YESTERDAY'S MAVENS, TODAY'S FOODIES

Yesterday's Mavens, Today's Foodies

TRADITIONS IN NORTHWEST JEWISH KITCHENS

A COLLECTION OF RECIPES AND STORIES
FROM THE

Washington State
JEWISH
HISTORICAL
SOCIETY

ISBN: 978-0-578-87475-3

Library of Congress Control Number: 2011915302

Printed in the United States of America

Cover design: Gordon Modin and Soundview Design Studio
Back cover photo: Dawn Lucrisia Photography
Book design: Soundview Design Studio

Washington State
JEWISH
HISTORICAL
SOCIETY

3801 E Mercer Way
Mercer Island, WA 98040
info@wsjhs.org • 206-774-2277

wsjhs.org
washingtonjewishmuseum.org

Washington State JEWISH HISTORICAL SOCIETY

10th Anniversary
Yesterday's Mavens, Today's Foodies

Commemoration of the 2nd Edition

It is so hard to believe that a decade ago, the Washington State Jewish Historical Society released the cookbook, *Yesterday's Mavens, Today's Foodies, Traditions in Northwest Jewish Kitchens (YMTF.)* It was a labor of love for all those who worked on the book. I particularly remember the fun and amazement as our dedicated group of volunteers joined with WSJHS staff to tirelessly gather 100's of recipes, sort through them, test and taste every single one of them. I think of all the people around Washington state we connected with and the folks who invited us into their homes to taste some of their most treasured recipes and share the rooted-in-history stories about them. We've been told that people sit down to read our cookbook as if it is a story book, which it truly is. That means the ultimate goal of *YMTF* was realized by creating this lasting piece of a culinary past for today and for generations to come.

Cindy Masin
Cookbook Chair

I remember working with Cindy Masin and her wonderful committee on the cookbook, now a decade ago. How time flies when preserving history! *YMTF* has a universal appeal, across generations and denominations and thus, I am not surprised that it is almost out of print and we are releasing the second and on demand printing edition. My family and I have used the cookbook as our go-to place for all recipes, as well as for the Jewish holidays. Every time I use a recipe, I usually get a history lesson along with my cooking preparation. In the past 10 years, I have learned to cook Sephardic foods, foreign to my upbringing and enjoyed new renditions from my own Ashkenazic background. I have "celebrated" holidays with our community's matriarchs and patriarchs and have learned the connections of whom is related to whom – it is endless. We live in such a connected community and state Jewishly and I am proud to be able to share in this history and do my part in assuring these stories will live on, in this cookbook's next edition and in our Washington Jewish Museum, our digital museum, where the cookbook page will live at: www.wsjhs.org/cookbook. Thanks to the writers and editors of the original cookbook edition and to those who helped with this second edition, as well. You have built history and on behalf of the Historical Society, your work is priceless.

Lisa Kranseler
WSJHS Executive Director

Contents

Foreword

When you're a lox-and-bagel Jew from Philadelphia, married to a fish-on-Friday Catholic from Chicago, living in a devoutly Christian town outside Seattle – 3,000 miles from the rest of your family – Jewish holidays tend to lose something in the translation. As do many of the other cultural touchstones that speak to our sense of place and tradition.

Yet, as we all know, home is where the heart is, and at the heart of every home is the kitchen. Though I was born and raised elsewhere, my heart is now firmly at home here in Washington State, thanks in large part to the warm embrace of the many Jewish friends I've come to know and love.

Among them are native Washingtonians like Cindy Masin, a member of a five-generation Seattle family, who has adopted my small "Jew-ish" family and introduced us to her own extended clan: superb cooks whose holiday tables we've gladly shared.

At their potluck festivities they've made it their business to show my young son the correct answer to two of the Four Questions: Question No. 1 (mine): "Do you have to be a James Beard Award-winning chef to cook like one?" (No.) And Question No. 2 (my husband's): "Isn't 'delicious Jewish food' an oxymoron?" (No!)

Cindy also introduced me to the Washington State Jewish Historical Society, whose mission is to collect, preserve, and disseminate the history of Washington's Jews. Together they cooked up the idea of the book you're holding in your hands: a very local culinary history rooted in the past but with an unwavering eye on a very delicious future.

If there's anything that binds a community, it's the foods we eat and the stories we tell as we share them. And here in the Northwest, Jewish foods and the people who love to create them continue to be a revelation to this longtime food writer.

As an Ashkenazi Jew who never heard the word Sephardim until I moved to Seattle, I was astonished to find a whole new world of dishes here I'd never tasted on my bubbie's table. (North African chicken with fennel and figs? Pass me a thigh!) Sure, this corner of the nation doesn't have the depth and breadth of the dreamy deli fare I was raised on, but it does have gefilte fish (homemade!) with fresh salmon, and did I mention Matzo Roca?

Now, with *Yesterday's Mavens, Today's Foodies* to broaden my palate and my repertoire, I feel an even greater sense of family: my Northwest family.

These are the scores of proud cooks and eaters, born as near as Mercer Island and as far as the island of Rhodes, who've contributed to this collection.

With them, I can rejoice in the memories behind classic dishes passed from one generation to the next and modern constructs sure to find a place in the canon of contemporary cookery.

With this book in hand, I am thrilled to find directions for preparing prakas and blintzes – just like the ones my mother made while my sisters and I watched *Here Come the Brides*, singing the theme-song along with heartthrob Bobby Sherman ("The bluest skies you've ever seen, in Seattle!").

I never imagined that one day I'd be cooking under those very skies, secure in the knowledge that as a Jew at home in the Northwest, I'll always live among family whose histories – in the kitchen and beyond its confines – will inevitably be intertwined with my own.

Nancy Leson
Seattle Times food and restaurant columnist

Introduction

YESTERDAY'S MAVENS, TODAY'S FOODIES: TRADITIONS IN NORTHWEST JEWISH KITCHENS

Food is culture, ritual, nourishment, and memory. Of late, food has become a modern obsession, an art form, an ethical-political statement, even a spectator sport. Food simultaneously defines and reflects culture, playing a key role in tradition's preservation and continuation.

The Washington State Jewish Historical Society is "dedicated to discovering, preserving, and disseminating the history of the Jews of Washington State." With the production of this community cookbook, we aim to reveal the culinary artifacts of Washington's Jews, simultaneously preserving these voices in amber and encouraging the pioneer spirit of innovation to play with and create new traditions.

The Jewish community in Washington is unique in that it comprises a blend of Ashkenazi and Sephardic Jews whose identities were little touched by the New York influence that came to define American Judaism. We can trace this adventurous spirit back to the founding fathers, many of whose family names have been passed down for more than a century and are proudly held by community members today. Unlike Jewish cookbooks that focus on one particular branch of ethnic Jewish cooking (often glorifying Eastern European staples over the gastronomic gifts of Jews from other regions), the book you are holding is remarkable in that it contains a cross section of Jewish culinary heritage, held together by a common dream and a shared space.

MAZOLA AND SCHMALTZ

It all began in 1845, when German immigrant Adolph Friedman stepped into Washington Territory. Waves of ambitious and entrepreneurial German and Eastern European immigrants ready to risk business on the frontier followed Friedman. By 1870 the territory had a Jewish governor, Edward S. Salomon, and by 1875 Seattle had its first (and only) Jewish mayor, Bailey Gatzert. The first Sephardic community members arrived in 1903 with the immigration of Solomon Calvo and Joseph Policar from Marmara and in 1904, Nessim Alhadeff from Rhodes.

Jewish communities blossomed in Olympia, Port Townsend, Tacoma, Bellingham, Spokane, and Seattle. In Seattle, the Turkish and Rhodesli immigrants moved in with the Eastern European Jews in the Yesler Way area, where about 85 percent of the Jewish community lived until World War I. By 1920 the Yesler Way neighborhood housed two Ashkenazi Orthodox synagogues and two Sephardi Orthodox synagogues, not to mention Jewish businesses, a cemetery, a B'nai B'rith chapter, social services, and schools. Sephardic families that immigrated at the turn of the century were instrumental in building the fish business in Seattle's historic Pike Place Market, and Calvo and Alhadeff founded what became Pacific Fish. But all was not harmonious. The European and Mediterranean Jews arrived to the Northwest with entirely different customs, even different languages: the Ashkenazi Jews spoke Yiddish, while the Sephardim spoke Ladino. Their liturgy, Hebrew pronunciation, dress, and food were entirely different. For many years, "mixed marriages" – that is, between Ashkenazi and Sephardi Jews – were discouraged and even shunned with great bitterness. In a Jewish version of Sharks versus Jets, Ashkenazi kids called the Sephardi kids "Mazola," and the Sephardi kids called the Ashkenazi kids "schmaltz," both names representing the kinds of fats their families traditionally cooked with. Since then, families descended from Seattle's first Jews have grown into dynasties that spread all over Seattle and beyond, and "intermarriage" is no longer shunned, but practiced regularly and joyfully.

MAVENS AND FOODIES

Thankfully, time and the adoption of an overarching American identity smoothed these conflicts over. But while we laugh and marvel at the trials our predecessors went through to simply date other Jews, our grafting onto American culture has posed another threat: the total dissolution of Jewish historical memory. How do we avoid fading into irrelevancy? How do we bridge the chasm between the immigrants of the old world with the children of the new global village?

Through food, of course. And more important, through the stories around the food. The stories included in *Yesterday's Mavens, Today's Foodies: Traditions in Northwest Jewish Kitchens* conjure images of grandmothers sitting down to chop liver in a wooden bowl by hand and mothers instructing daughters to treat dough gently, "like a baby's bottom." Others offer a glimpse into the human condition during wartime. Many stories invoke the spirits of the deceased, who seem to be present when their favorite dish is recreated. Others see their legacy unfold as they teach their children and grandchildren the techniques of a sacred family recipe.

When we began thinking about mavens and foodies, we unconsciously divided them along age and gender lines. Most simplistically, mavens are the grandmothers, foodies are the grandchildren. The older mavens create the timeless traditional dishes, while the young foodies invent culinary curiosities. But as we sifted through hundreds of recipes spanning ages, places, and backgrounds, we found ourselves struggling with this basic understanding. To help, we turn to some definitions.

The word "maven" comes from the Hebrew verb "lehaveen," "to understand." This word implies wisdom, intuition, and cognizance. Mavens are "ones who understand" food and the kitchen. The term "maven" almost imbues the cook with a sense of spiritual intuition, maybe a deeper knowledge of what food does for the soul. "Foodie" is a new word coined in American dialect, meaning someone who is enthusiastic or passionate for food. Foodies can take many forms: They may love experimenting with obscure ingredients.

They may grow their own vegetables and raise their own chickens and belong to a co-op. They may never use the kitchen and relate to food solely through the dining experience. "Foodie" crosses gender lines and stresses a sense of adventure and passion.

In this light, many of our contributors are both mavens and foodies. At any age, they connect with the spiritual energy of the kitchen and with new innovative creations. We have older contributors who share inspired new delicacies and young contributors who return to their roots. Some recipes honor the past, others create the future. The definitions are fluid and subjective.

THEN AND NOW

Our recipes hearken back to migration tales, war stories, pioneering days, and the previous eras in our family histories. Sensory memories, especially the sense of smell, are evoked and transport us into another time, another family, to another table that somehow feels like home. Descriptions are as rich as a creamy noodle pudding – at once we are surrounded by trees dripping sticky, sweet plums in Germany, under a canopy of stars on Whidbey Island, crammed into a kitchen packed with women and a gorgeous spread of Sephardic delicacies.

Madeline Caston Sherman explains that, "Hospitality was a way of life in the early twentieth century, as there were no televisions, cineplexes, or computers, and people frequently visited each other without the need of an invitation. For these occasions, Turkish coffee, cookies, and homemade sweets were served. Sephardic kitchens were the place where sumptuous treats were labored over with love."

Debra Schwartz, Gail Alexander, and Steve Schwartz remember: "Whenever we set our tables for the holidays or special dinners with Mom's beautiful green glasses, Aunt Minnie's fine china, our grandmother Sarah Golombeck's candelabra, and Mom's linens, we can almost feel the arms of those from generations past wrapped around us."

These sensory experiences may be as close as we get to the past. However, we want to emphasize the traditions continually being made that will be passed down with as much love to the next generations. In fact, we can trace a thread between several multi-generational families represented on these pages. For instance, Molly and Jerry Cone submit recipes along with their granddaughter, Dani Cone, who uses a family pie recipe at her own pie shop, High Five Pie. Both Rivy Poupko Kletenik and her daughter, Gilah, share traditional recipes from their festive tables. Becky Benaroya's mavenly recipe complements her granddaughter Brooke's decidedly foodie dishes. Karen Hudesman and Sharon Lott contribute recipes alongside their married children, Andrea (Karen's daughter) and Jordan (Sharon's son).

It's impossible to know which recipes will come to define our future traditions. Whether we end up using Mazola or schmaltz or a drizzle of truffle oil, we hope the awareness of how it all began will guide us in perpetuating our heritage.

Acknowledgments

On behalf of the Washington State Jewish Historical Society, we would like to thank its members and friends who contributed so much to *Yesterday's Mavens, Today's Foodies: Traditions in Northwest Jewish Kitchens.*

Hundreds of people have touched the production of this book. (please see our Acknowledgment List on pages xiv-xv.) Mavens lovingly shared recipes written on splattered, tattered, and faded cards and pages in journals, and foodies have virtually submitted their entries by way of their smart phones or computers. We received over 400 recipes from all around Washington State for this project. We appreciate the thought and time that went into the selection of the recipes submitted. Can you imagine the difficult task of deciding which ones to actually put in the cookbook?

We had many recipes for the same traditional favorites: gefilte fish, chopped liver, borekas, biscochos, kugels, and briskets. We were simply unable to put them all in the cookbook, but your stories, in your own voices, have been just as meaningful to us and we have included them wherever possible.

Thanks go to our cookbook committee, which has been a fantastic sounding board, as well as to our story and recipe submitters, testers and tasters, editorial and content advisors, copy editors and proofreaders, and our generous financial supporters, who have **all** been valuable ingredients in assuring the quality of this community treasure. To those of you who welcomed us into your homes to share special meals and allowed us the privilege of looking at your precious diaries and journals replete with family stories and recipes, many thanks.

There is a phrase we hear all the time: "We couldn't have done it without you." We surely could not have taken on – and completed – this project without Carol Starin. *Yesterday's Maven's, Today's Foodies* would not have come to fruition were it not for her encouragement, calm, collaboration, breadth of community knowledge, passion for genealogy, willingness to listen, and her love of a great story. Carol planned a plethora of fun and educational classes and dine-arounds, and with Iantha Sidell, raised the dollars necessary to underwrite the publishing of this book.

Special thanks to the staff at the Washington State Jewish Historical Society, Lisa Kranseler for her leadership, and Lori Weinberg Ceyhun for her participation in receiving and chronicling the recipes and stories and being the keeper of the volunteer and donor lists. Emily Keeler Alhadeff has been our project manager for *Yesterday's Mavens, Today's Foodies*. She is also a gifted writer who has woven together all the threads of the stories to create the wonderful introductions for the book and each chapter section, with the editorial help of Cynthia Shifrin. We also thank The Jewish Federation of Greater Seattle and *JTNews* for their tremendous support.

The committee is forever grateful to Andrea Lott, (author of her own cookbook, *Dining In Seattle: Past and Present*) who put in hundreds of hours as an editorial consultant, typist, and copy-editor to keep this project moving forward. Where would we be without her? Andrea, Anna Brown, Linda Morgan, Cherie Tucker, Emily Keeler Alhadeff, and Carol Starin devoted weeks and weeks to copy-editing and proofreading the entire book. Andrea, Emily, Sherry Benaroya, and Brooke Benaroya Dickson developed a style guide for our typists, Andrea, Robyn Anderson, Morrene Jacobson, and Laurie Koehler. Gayle Carrol entered and managed all the index listings, and Marilyn Brody tirelessly and constantly updated the spreadsheet of all the recipes. Thanks to Katherine Scharhon and Hannah Cordes for posing for the back cover photo. We couldn't have done it without you.

Kathy Fishman and Doreen Alhadeff stepped up to coordinate all the testings and tastings that led to recipes being chosen for the cookbook. To the testers and tasters who were entreated to "follow the recipes exactly" – and did as they made their way through over 400 recipes – and to Kathy and Doreen, without whom none of that would have happened, thank you, thank you.

We also thank Elliott Wolf, our publisher, who since the beginning of this project, asked the tough questions and guided us on the path to accomplishing our goals.

To Nancy Leson, *Seattle Times* food and restaurant columnist, foreword writer, and new member of the Masin family, thank you so much for agreeing to write the foreword for this cookbook.

Last but not least, thanks to all our many family members and friends whose great advice, patience, understanding, and love saw us through the creation of *Yesterday's Mavens, Today's Foodies: Traditions in Northwest Jewish Kitchens.* Your support has been truly invaluable.

Cookbook Committee
Yesterday's Mavens, Today's Foodies: Traditions in Northwest Jewish Kitchens
Cindy Masin, Chairperson

We express our deep appreciation to the following for their generosity in underwriting the publication of our cookbook, *Yesterday's Mavens, Today's Foodies: Traditions in Northwest Jewish Kitchens.*

"So, have a nosh."

MICHELE AND STAN ROSEN

"Enjoy!"

MARLEEN AND KENNY ALHADEFF, JT NEWS, JEWISH FEDERATION OF GREATER SEATTLE, SHARON AND MARTY LOTT AND FAMILY, ALFRED AND TILLIE SHEMANSKI FOUNDATION

"It is a sin to throw it away...so it shouldn't be wasted."

MARILYN AND DICK BRODY, CINDY AND BOB MASIN AND FAMILY, IANTHA AND STAN SIDELL, CAROL STARIN, SHEILA AND CRAIG STERNBERG

"Eat a little something."

QUALITY FOOD CENTERS, BETSY AND JASON SCHNEIER, BARBARA AND STUART SULMAN AND FAMILY (SCOTT SULMAN, SCOTT, CARIN, RYAN AND LUKE JACOBSON)

"Come on. Live a little."

SHERRY AND LARRY BENAROYA, MAUREEN AND JOEL BENOLIEL, JEFFREY B.COOPERSMITH, STEFANIE SNOW, MATTHEW COOPERSMITH AND JOSHUA COOPERSMITH, SANDY AND KEN GLASS, GENA AND SONNY GORASHT, NICK AND MICHELE KELLER, JACKIE AND SKIP KOTKINS, RALPH AND ESTHER MAIMON, RABBI JIM AND JULIE MIREL, ANN NIEDER, FIL AND JANET ROSE, DEBORAH AND DOUGLAS ROSEN, JUDY AND KERMIT ROSEN, RUTH SASSOON, GOLDIE AND DON SILVERMAN, BOBBIE AND MICHEL STERN, CARLYN KOCH STEINER, MARCIE AND DAVE STONE, CINDY AND BOB STRAUSS, HELEN STUSSER, GOLDIE TOBIN

"Eat already!"

DEANNA MOINESTER ALBERT, GAIL AND BOB ALEXANDER, ALPHAGRAPHICS, TAMAR BENZIKRY-STERN AND RONNIE STERN, LOU BERG, JANET AND JIM BLUE, ANNA AND JOE BROWN, JOEL BUXBAUM, INEZ AND LIOR CASPI, DIANE AND MIKE CHEIFETZ, JERRY AND DIANE COHN, STEVE COOPERSMITH AND TONY SCHIERLING, LILLY DEJAEN, JOYCE ROSEN DICKHAUT, JULIE FAISON, LINDA AND GARY FELDMAN, KATHY AND MARK FISHMAN, KAREN MAYERS GAMORAN FOUNDATION, CAROLE AND BOB GOLDBERG, DENNIS GOLDSTEIN AND ROBIN ROGEL-GOLDSTEIN, DARCY GOODMAN AND TOM LEAVITT, JANET GRAY AND BRAD RIND, JOE AND LILA GREENGARD, LESLEY AND JEFF GROSVENOR, LEATRICE GUTMANN, CAROL AND ANDY HARRIS, ELLEN AND JERRY HENDIN, KAREN HUDESMAN AND DON STARK, ALBERT ISRAEL, SUSAN AND HANK KAPLAN, KLINE GALLAND CENTER, LISA AND KENNY KRANSELER, MARILYN AND BRIAN KREMEN, PATTY AND JONATHAN LAZARUS, HERB LIPMAN, PAUL AND JENNIFER MALAKOFF, DAVID, ANNE, GRANT AND ELLA MASIN, LAURA AND BRAD MILLER, LINDA AND MIKE MORGAN, CINDY AND MOE MUSCATEL, SUE AND HOWARD ROBBOY, FRANCES ROGERS, ALAN AND LESLIE ROSEN, BETTY AND RANDY RUBENSTEIN, STEPHEN SADIS, JUDY AND JOE SCHOCKEN, RABBIS JONATHAN AND BETH SINGER, WENDY AND MICHAEL SPEKTOR, MIMI STERNBERG AND BILLY HOWARD, DORIS STIEFEL, STOPSKY'S DELICATESSEN, SAM AND SUE TARICA, ELISE TOPP, NINA AND RODNEY WALDBAUM, RUTH WINSTON

4 CULTURE

WE APPRECIATE THE CONTINUED SUPPORT OF 4 CULTURE.

THE WSJHS THANKS THE ISAAC N. ALHADEFF FOUNDATION FOR THEIR SUPPORT OF THE SECOND EDITION.

We gratefully acknowledge the following people. Without their support, this project would have never been possible.

Steve Adler
Gail Alexander
Doreen Alhadeff
Emily Keeler Alhadeff
Jeanie Alhadeff
Joan Mandas Alhadeff
Kenny Alhadeff
Marleen Alhadeff
Roly Alhadeff
Rachel Almeleh
Amanda Lyon
Judith Amiel
Robyn Anderson
Irene Arron
Brenda Atkin
Amanda Azous
Janti Baroh
Kathie Barokas
Del Baron
Edie Bean
Susan Beardsley
Dorothy Becker
Lynette Benaltabe
Becky Benaroya
Sherry Benaroya
Berdine Bender
Maureen Benoliel
Gloria Bensussen
Shelley Bensussen
Louise Chiprut Berman
Karen Binder
Jan Block
Terry Bloom
Frankie Bookey
Bel Borromeo
Bobbi Bridge
Rabbi Dan Bridge
Dick Brody
Marilyn Brody
Anna Brown
Deb Brownstein
Rodrigo Caamano
Wendy Caamano
Marcia Calvo
Gayle Carrol
Inez Caspi
Lian Caspi
Lori Weinberg Ceyhun
Karen Chachkes
Diane Cheifetz
Michael Cheifetz
Esther Chiprut
Miriam Coates
Carolyn Cohen
Jill Cohen
Diane Cohn
Dani Cone
Jerry Cone
Karen Cone
Molly Cone
Hannah Cordes
Beth Cordova
Nancy Corning
Rabbi Avroham David
Marjorie Danz
Beverly DeJaen
Lilly DeJaen
Joyce Dickhaut
Brooke Benaroya Dickson
Diane Douglas
Howard Droker
Julia Niebuhr Eulenberg
Julie Faison
Blair Feehan
Linda Feldman
Beth Fine
Debbie Fishman
Kathy Fishman
Mark Fishman
Sarah Fishman
Todd Fishman
Deb Freedman
Lucy Friedman
Patty Friedman
Josh Furman
Jon Fuson
Marlene Fuson
Barrie Galanti
Joel Gamoran
Karen Gamoran
Joan Garden
Sandy Glass
Lois Kaplan Glickman
Joanne Glosser
Carole Goldberg
Jackie Goldfarb
Darcy Goodman
Carol Gown
Beverly Grashin
Beverly Greenberg
Joe Greengard
Lila Greengard
Jeff Grosvenor
Lesley Masin Grosvenor
Leatrice Gutmann
Lea Hamlin
Enid Hammer
Carol Harris
Cynthia Flash Hemphill
Shannon Frisch Herman
Toddy Horowitz
Karen Hudesman
Leslie Huppin
Kim Haas Isaac
Jane Isenberg
Albert Israel
Daisy Israel
Karen Israel
Carin Jacobson
Morrene Jacobson
Leah Jaffee
Camille Jassny
Jo Jassny
Luetta Jermulowske
Jewish Federation of Greater Seattle
JTNews
Tina Lippman Kahn
Lita Kaplan
Janice Kaplan-Klein
Julie Katz
Laurie Katz
Judith Kay
Frances Keller
Michele Keller
Jamie Kezner
Rabbi Yohanna Kinberg
Chaya Kinberg

Gilah Kletenik
Rivy Poupko Kletenik
Laurie Koehler
Bob Kollack
Linda Kollack
Jackie Kotkins
Kenny Kranseler
Lisa Kranseler
Marilyn Kremen
Eileen Kulman
Loretta Kuznetz
Tina Lamb
Darcy Leavitt
Dorothy Lederman
Margaret Lemberg
Joan Lerner
Nancy Leson
Robin Leventhal
Jan Lewis
Rhoda Lewis
Steve Lewis
Esther Lipson
Andrea Lott
Jordan Lott
Sharon Lott
Wendy Lynne
Joel Magalnick
Esther Maimon
Jeanne Maimon
Natalie Malin
Mary Anne Stusser Martin
Anne Masin
Bob Masin
Cindy Masin
David Masin
Fred Maslan
Debbie Goldberg Menashe
Miriam Meyerson
Pip Meyerson
Katherine Zinger Miller
Laura Miller
Dan Mintz
Linda Morgan
Margaret Mosholder
Cindy Muscatel
Gloria Newman
Ann Nieder
Mary Noble
Esther Normand
Eugene Normand
Marjorie Offer
Bill Oseran
Jean Oseran
Sylvia Oseran
Sandra Ostroff
Joy Paltiel
Leslie Person
Roz Poll
Randy Pollock
Jane Preuss
Sharon Prosser
Esther Quint
Janet Reis
Nancy Resnik
Jack Richlen
Bernice Rind
Sue Robboy
Bob Rogers
Frances Rogers
Joyce Lighter Rogers
Fil Rose
Janet Rose
Ken Rose
Laurie Rose
Shirley Rose
Judy Rosen
Leslie Rosen
Michele Rosen
Phyllis Rosen
Rabbi Jay Rosenbaum
Norma Rosenthal
Sue Robboy
Betty Rubenstein
Deanne Seinfeld Rubinstein
Gladys Rubinstein
Esther Sadis
Stephen Sadis
Jeff Sanderson
David Sanford
Joani Diskin Saran
Faye Sarkowsky
Ruth Sassoon
Katherine Scharhon
Betsy R. Schneier
Judy Schocken
Ruth Schocken
Bev Schoenfeld
Arlene Mosler Schuster
Debra Schwartz
Joanne Schwartz
Ken Schwartz
Steve Schwartz
Marcia Shahon
Adele Sharaga
Madeleine Caston Sherman
Susie Sherman
Cynthia Shifrin
Marilyn Sidel
Iantha Sidell
Alice Siegal
Goldie Silverman
Lauren Silvernail
Michelle Sloan
Lynn Snyder
Joanne Sobel
Mark Solomon
Frieda Sondland
Mimi Sorkin
Wendy Spektor
Lucy Almeleh Spring
Carol Starin
Geoff Starin
Carlyn Koch Steiner
Bobbie Stern
Craig Sternberg
Sheila Sternberg
Doris Stiefel
Marcie Stone
Cindy Stratiner
Gary Stratiner
Cindy Fein Strauss
Helen Stusser
Isabel Stusser
Laura Stusser-McNeill
Barbara Sulman
Ruth Sulman
Michele Tesler
Lennard Thal
Goldie Tobin
Elise Topp
Nina Waldbaum
Lilly Warnick
Diane Warshal
Lynn Wartnik
Tony Wartnik
Amy Wasser-Simpson
Lee Weinstein
Jackie Williams
Ruth Winston
Elliott Wolf
Barbara Wolf
Beverly Wolfers
Dana Wootten
Bonnie Zell

as of September, 9, 2011

Jewish Federation
OF GREATER SEATTLE
Connecting Jewish Lives. Strengthening Community.

It is with great pleasure that the Jewish Federation of Greater Seattle supports publication of this delicious cookbook filled with the recipes that nourish our lives.

We are proud of the rich and diverse traditions of our Jewish community and applaud the Washington State Jewish Historical Society for helping keep those traditions alive and well in our kitchens and on our tables.

Food has long been an important way for the generations to connect and to share family history. The schmoozing involved in preparing and eating a meal is an important part of our Jewish ritual, providing a strong bond between family and friends.

Our Ethnic Flavors cooking program brought to our community extraordinary cooks and amazing meals from the diverse cultures living in Kiryat Malachi and Hof Ashkelon, our partnership region in Israel. This was a shining example of how food connects all members of the Jewish community, regardless of where our families originated.

This cookbook will enrich the lives of our Jewish community members, strengthening the links between generations. The Jewish Federation builds and sustains a vibrant Jewish community, locally and abroad, for all Jews. Projects such as this cookbook enhance home and synagogue life, creating opportunities to instill our Jewish values with the flavors of our ancestors.

Congratulations to the WSJHS on publication of this book. We look forward to many more years of helping you connect your passions to meaningful impact in our Jewish community.

Mazel Tov!

Richard Fruchter, President & CEO
Jewish Federation of Greater Seattle

TIPS & TRICKS:

- ❖ You will notice sidebars with this heading as you read through *Yesterday's Mavens, Today's Foodies.* They are meant to guide you toward possible short cuts, substitutions, additional ingredient options, equipment necessities and so on.
- ❖ The greatest tip we can possibly give our readers is to read every recipe in it's entirety before starting to make it. That way you will know what to purchase at the store as well as what is in store for you as you prepare the recipe.

~*Yesterday's Maven's, Today's Foodies*
Traditions in Northwest Jewish Kitchens
Editorial Committee

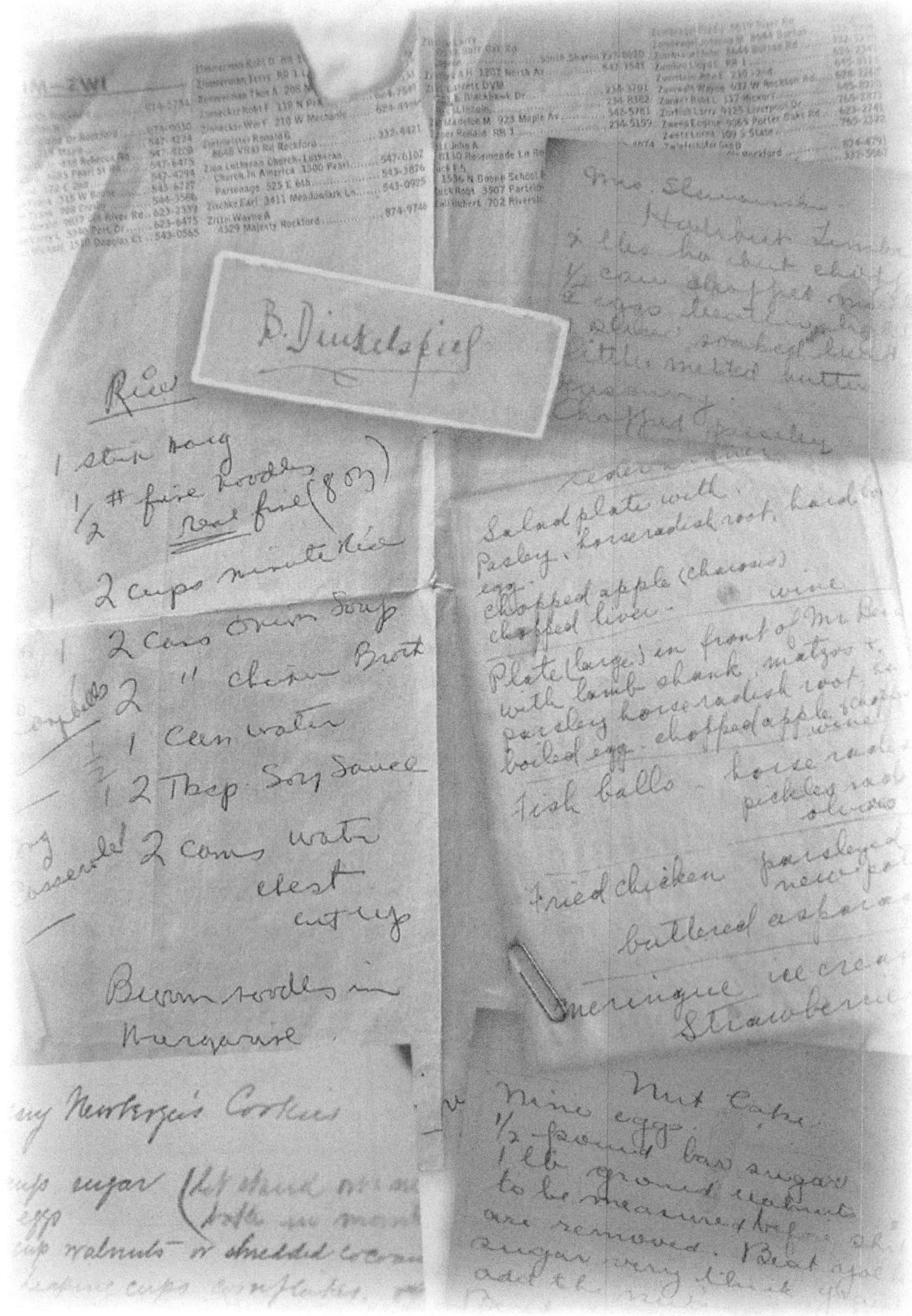
B. Dinkelspiel
Rice
Nut Cake

Noshes and Mezzes

The concept of the appetizer – that prelude to a meal replete with savory finger foods that, as we so often realize a moment too late, could in fact stand in for the meal itself – appears across cultures and reaches deep into history. In the Middle East this course may be known as *mezze*, in Italy *antipasti*, in Spain *tapas* or else as small plates, or, as many Jews know, a little nosh.

While chopped liver spread on a cracker and popped in the mouth is a nostalgic nosh of choice among many, especially older, Ashkenazi Jews, our Sephardic community members weighed in heavily with warm anecdotes about the finger foods prepared by female family members gathered in the kitchen, "a place where lively conversation mixed with the aroma of *boyos* baking."

Sharon Lott shares a vivid reflection of the many Friday afternoons passed with her Sephardic extended family in the kitchen, where up to ten women would huddle together over coffee, homemade grape leaves, fresh vegetables, and piles of food in a scene that calls to her mind a rich still life painting.

As we shall see from the variety of recipes in this chapter, culture and era affect the dynamic of the appetizer. Chopped liver is lightened up, mayonnaise is reduced, a painstaking knish recipe is reinvented with instant potatoes and puff pastry. Signature American concoctions, like Todd Fishman's spicy-sweet salami appetizer or Andrea Lott's cowboy salsa, are especially well-suited to the margaritas and mojitos. The inclusion of cocktails alone signifies an American influence, the popularity of the "cocktail hour."

While traditional recipes are modified with the times and while fresh creations constantly hit the dining room table, the shadow of our ancestors never recedes too far. Molly Cone poignantly expresses this idea in describing her relationship to chopped liver: Just the act of writing out her chopped liver recipe conjures the image of her grandmother preparing the dish with a bowl and a blade, long before the days of the Cuisinart. And yet looking forward, she sees the joy on her own granddaughter's face as she takes that first bite, that same joy she felt as a granddaughter herself.

TIDBIT:
Borekas, those savory pastries signature to Sephardic cuisine, trace back to the Ottoman Empire and manifest in virtually every country's cuisine from Albania to Israel and beyond. Borekas even inspired an entire genre of film: Melodramatic, Sephardic-themed "borekas films" are Israel's version of spaghetti westerns. But borekas aren't the only Jewish appetizer to claim fame. The Jewish American expression, "what am I, chopped liver?" likely came about because chopped liver was always a side dish on the Shabbat table, never the main attraction.

NOSHES AND MEZZES

THE BEST CHOPPED LIVER IN TOWN

Carole Goldberg

"This recipe for 'The Best Chopped Liver in Town' comes from Sonny Gorasht and the rest of the family. It has become a staple at all our family and holiday dinners. Since my husband does not really like liver, I had to make adjustments to my mother's original recipe so that my chopped liver did not taste too 'livery.' And if I don't make it for all the holiday dinners, there is a major rebellion by all in attendance. I still use Bubbie Gorasht's original hand-grinder from Calgary, which seems to be the key to getting the perfect consistency."

Serves 4 to 6

1 pound beef or calf's liver
4 ounces kosher chicken fat, divided
Pepper
Garlic powder
Seasoned salt
Paprika
1 to 1½ large onions, sliced
6 eggs, hard-boiled, cooled, and peeled

Put the liver on the top of a broiler pan. Brush with 1 ounce of the chicken fat and season well with pepper, garlic powder, and seasoned salt.

Broil the liver on high until cooked on one side. Turn the liver over and season the other side. Continue broiling until the liver is well done; be sure there is no pink inside. Set aside to cool.

In a separate sauté pan, add the remaining 3 tablespoons of the chicken fat and season with the pepper, garlic powder, seasoned salt, and paprika. Sauté the onions in the seasoned fat.

Mash the hard-boiled eggs very well by hand or in food processor and transfer to a bowl. Chop the sautéed onions in the food processor. Add the onions to the mashed eggs and mix well.

Grind the broiled liver. Add it to the egg mixture and blend well; taste and adjust seasonings if needed. Refrigerate overnight to allow flavors to blend.

TIPS & TRICKS:

- Make this dish a day ahead to give the flavors a chance to blend.
- Serve with crackers, rye bread, or challah.
- This recipe is good for 4 to 6 people as an appetizer. It can be doubled to serve 8 to 12 people. A little extra is never a bad thing, and I'm sure someone will want to take a doggie bag home.

FAUX CHOPPED LIVER

Kathy Fishman

"My sister-in-law makes this appetizer before holiday meals. It has been a family favorite, especially for those who are not true liver fans!"

Makes 4 cups

1 teaspoon vegetable oil
2 tablespoons butter, room temperature
3 medium onions, chopped
2 eggs, hard-boiled
1 14-ounce can green peas, drained
¾ cup walnuts, toasted
1 can dried French onions, as a garnish
Party rye bread

In a food processor, blend the oil, butter, onions, hard-boiled eggs, peas, and walnuts until smooth. Pour into a bowl and refrigerate overnight.

When ready to serve, sprinkle the top with the French onions and serve with party rye.

"My mother's name is Ruth Elaine Jacobson Katz, and she and my father, Seymour Katz, a physician and surgeon, moved to Waukegan, Illinois, on January 1, 1937. This was six months after they wed in Chicago, Illinois. I grew up in Waukegan, where my mother was famous for her chopped liver. A local popular restaurant asked for her recipe so that they could serve it. The healthy secret was that the onions were not rendered in chicken fat."

~ Marjorie Offer

CHOPPED LIVER PÂTÉ

Molly Cone

"As I write out this recipe, I think of my grandmother sitting on a kitchen chair with a wooden bowl on her lap and a small chopping blade doing what my Cuisinart does for me today. But my recipe is not exactly the same as my grandmother's. I use chicken livers instead of beef liver and olive oil instead of rendered chicken fat. What is the same is the delight on my granddaughter, Sara's, face as she savors the first dab of the chicken liver pate on a cracker. It is exactly what I felt on every first taste of my grandmother's chopped liver when I was the granddaughter."

Makes about 2 cups

8 ounces chicken livers
1 small onion, sliced into thin rings
2 tablespoons plus 1 teaspoon olive oil
1 egg, hard-boiled
¼ to ½ teaspoon salt
⅛ coarsely ground black pepper
Pinch of cayenne powder
2 teaspoons parsley, finely chopped, as a garnish

Rinse and drain the chicken livers.

Sauté the onions in 2 tablespoons of the olive oil until golden. Push onions to the edge of the pan. Sauté the chicken livers in the center of the pan, until well cooked and tender. Transfer the sautéed onions and liver to the food processor. Add the hard-boiled egg and process until lightly blended. Add the remaining teaspoon of olive oil, salt, and pepper until finely blended. Adjust for proper seasoning. Add the cayenne pepper.

Mound the chopped liver in a small bowl. Sprinkle with the parsley and refrigerate.

CHOPPED LIVER LITE

Lilly Warnick

"As a young bride of 19 in the early 50s – straight from the sorority – I had no cooking experience and relied solely on my mother-in-law, Phreda Soss Warnick, for recipes, particularly those for the Jewish holidays. At the time, chopped liver was a favorite and often served as an appetizer or even as a first course, mounded on a bed of lettuce with radish and tomato slices. Schmaltz (rendered chicken fat) held the ingredients together. Knowing now that schmaltz is a 'killer,' I finally discovered a version that tastes equally as good as the original recipe. 'Chopped Liver Lite' sounds like an oxymoron, but it is delicious."

Makes 4 to 5 cups

½ pound chicken livers
Kosher salt
2 tablespoon vegetable oil
2 medium onions, chopped
1 15-ounce can chickpeas, drained and rinsed
4 to 5 tablespoons chicken broth
1 egg, hard-boiled and grated
Salt and freshly ground pepper

Preheat the broiler. Put the livers on a foil-lined pan and sprinkle with the salt. Broil for 3 minutes, about 3 inches from the heat, until the top is light brown. Flip and broil for an additional 3 more minutes, until cooked through or no longer pink. Cool slightly.

In a large skillet over medium-low heat, sauté the onions in the oil until completely soft.

Grind the chickpeas and 4 tablespoons of the chicken broth in a food processor. Transfer to a bowl.

Add the sautéed onions to the food processor and pulse until just blended. Return the chickpeas to the food processor and pulse to blend with the onions, adding the remaining tablespoon of broth, if necessary. **Do not over-pulse**. Transfer to a bowl and mix in the egg. Season with salt and pepper and serve chilled.

TUNA PÂTÉ

Gloria Newman

Makes 4 cups

1 8-ounce package cream cheese, softened
2 tablespoons chili sauce
2 tablespoons parsley, chopped
1 teaspoon dried minced onion
½ teaspoon Tabasco sauce
2 7-ounce cans tuna, drained
Crackers, for serving

Grease a 4-cup mold.

Blend together the cream cheese, chili sauce, parsley, onion, Tabasco sauce, and tuna and pack into a 4-cup mold. Chill for at least 3 hours. Unmold and serve with crackers.

HELEN'S CHOPPED HERRING

Sandra Ostroff

"This is our family's favorite appetizer and my signature dish – even my grandchildren all love it! I make it for Rosh Hashanah and all year round for company. This was my mother's recipe, and I'm not sure where it came from, but it's a classic dish. It's great with crackers, or I eat it straight off of a spoon!"

Makes 4 cups

2 pieces challah or rye bread without crust, dried (baked in a 200° oven for 2 to 4 hours, being careful not to brown)
1 small granny smith apple, peeled, cored, and chopped into chunks
1 medium onion (sweet if possible)
3 eggs, hard-boiled
1 teaspoon sugar
12 ounce jar pickled herring, drained

Using a food processor, pulse the bread until it is very fine. Add the apple, then the onion and chop. Add the egg, sugar, and herring and mix until desired consistency.

TIPS & TRICKS:

- The order of mixing is important because you want the bread to be pulverized and the apple, onion, and egg to be finely chopped.
- The herring keeps well in the fridge for a long time and freezes well. It is easy to make and the ingredients are available year round.

BOREKAS DE AROZ

Lucille Almeleh Spring

"At the age of 4, Victoria Almeleh and her family moved from the Isle of Rhodes to Montgomery, Alabama, for a safer and better life. When she graduated from high school, her mother sent her to Seattle as a graduation gift. She remembers her mother saying, 'Go find your mazel.*' It wasn't too long before her cousin Nessim Peha introduced her to one of his young employees, Pinhas Almeleh. She had found her* mazel.

"My mother knew it was not her cooking that won the heart of Pinhas. When she moved to Seattle, cooking was a bit of a mystery to her. But she learned from the best: Senora Sadis, Behora Israel, and Serena Mossafer, her cousins. Lucy remembers her mother telling her, 'I had to watch them very carefully because they didn't have any measurements written down. I became a master at turning their pinches into measurements. I soon became good at making Sephardic specialties like quesado de spinaca, borekas de aroz, *and* kivteh de prasa.*' As I joined my mother in the kitchen, we made sure to meticulously measure and write down ingredients, so all the recipes could be passed down to my children and grandchildren.*

"Because my mother went through the depression years, she became a 'recycler' long before it was fashionable. As a result, she used the unprinted side of mail and cards and invitations to write her recipes on. I could so determine the date she wrote down her recipes by the date of the event on the other side.

"My mother was one of the few Sephardic women in Seattle who made borekas de aroz, *as most women made, and still make,* borekas de patata *(with potato) or sometimes* borekas de calavasa *(with pumpkin or squash). My mother's recipe uses a 'gomu' (filling) of rice, eggs, and cheese. I think they are much more savory and richer-bodied."*

Makes 24 to 30 borekas

Filling:
4 cups water
2 cups raw, short-grain rice
Pinch of salt
8 extra-large eggs
16 ounces Romano cheese, grated
16 ounces cottage cheese

Bring the water to a boil. Add the rice and salt. Cook according to the package directions. When done, transfer the rice to a large bowl and cool.

When completely cool, add the eggs, one at a time, then both the Romano and cottage cheeses, and mix well. Refrigerate the mixture.

Dough:
6½ cups flour
Pinch of salt
1¼ cup oil
1 cup ice water

Sift the flour into a large bowl. Whisk in the salt then stir in the oil and the ice water. Mix the dough well and let it sit for 1 hour.

For Brushing and Sprinkling:
1 egg, beaten
½ cup each Romano and Parmesan, blended

Preheat the oven to 375°. Line a baking sheet with parchment paper.

Gather and roll the dough into balls about the size of a walnut. Temporarily place the balls in a well-oiled, shallow baking sheet with sides. Roll out one ball at a time into a circle approximately 3 inches in diameter. Place a scant tablespoon of the filling in the middle of the circle and fold in half. Either flute the edges, or with the tines of a fork, press the edges together. Repeat the process until all the balls are rolled out and filled.

Place the borekas on the baking sheet. Brush with the egg, then sprinkle with the cheeses.

Bake for 20 to 25 minutes, 10 to 15 minutes on the bottom shelf then 10 minutes or so on the top shelf.

"Our family serves borekas every year to break the fast on Yom Kippur. Four generations of my family plus dear friends gather each year to make this delicacy. Our dedicated group of bakers range in age from 6 to 86 and represent diverse religious beliefs and ethnicities. The morning is filled with laughter, appreciation, and anticipation of a delicious end to a day of fasting."

~ Beverly Greenberg

BOREKAS

Esther Sadis

Makes 36 borekas

Dough:
1 cup oil
¾ cup ice water
1 teaspoon salt
3½ to 4 cups flour

Mix the oil, water, and salt. Add 3½ cups of the flour to start. Mix with a spoon or your hands. Break off a portion of dough and roll into walnut-sized balls or, for larger borekas, golf ball-sized balls. Set aside on a baking sheet lined with parchment paper.

Filling:
7 medium potatoes, peeled and quartered
6 tablespoons butter
2 eggs, beaten
1 cup feta cheese plus a bit extra, crumbled
1 cup Romano or Parmesan cheese (or a mixture of the two), plus more for sprinkling
Pinch of salt
1 egg, beaten, or oil, for brushing

Boil the potatoes until done. Drain the water and mash the potatoes while they are hot. Add the butter, eggs, feta, Romano and/or Parmesan cheese, and salt. Mix well, then cool.

Preheat the oven to 375°. Line a baking sheet with parchment paper.

To assemble the borekas, roll one piece of dough at a time into a 4-inch circle. Put a heaping tablespoon of filling on the circle and fold the dough over, crimping the edges with the tines of a fork. Brush the tops with the beaten egg or oil. Sprinkle with Romano cheese, as Romano won't burn.

Place the borekas on the baking sheet. Bake for 25 to 30 minutes, until brown.

TIPS & TRICKS:

- The filling recipe makes twice the amount needed for this dough.
- Make the potato filling the day before if desired and bring it to room temperature for 30 minutes before filling.
- The borekas can be made and frozen without baking. Freeze on a baking sheet then place standing up in a foil- or wax paper-lined box until ready to bake.

CHEESE BOREKAS

Peggy Maimon

"Everything my mother, Becky Mutal, cooked or baked was delicious and so, so beautiful. For instance, when she was teaching her girls how to make bulemas, she told us to treat the dough gently, like a baby's bottom. The same held true for her borekas and all that she tackled. Her food was amazing. She took so much pride in everything she did. My mother loved people and made so many friends wherever she went. To this day I still have so many people who want to share stories about my mother. She was so beautiful, vivacious, compassionate, kind, and loving, with an amazing spirit. Her family meant everything to her, and it showed with how much she loved watching us all enjoy the food she created."

Makes about 30 borekas

Filling:
3/4 cup water
1/3 cup milk
1/4 teaspoon salt
1/2 teaspoon margarine or butter
1 1/4 cup Potato Buds
1/2 cup feta cheese, crumbled
1/4 cup Romano cheese, grated
1/4 cup Parmesan cheese, grated
2 eggs plus a possible 2 additional eggs, for fluffiness

The filling should be made first and be allowed to cool. Bring the water and milk to a boil, then add the salt and margarine. Remove the pan from the heat and add the potato buds, feta, Romano and Parmesan cheeses, and eggs. Cool.

Dough:
1/2 cup oil
3/8 cup ice water
Pinch of salt
1 7/8 cup flour
1 egg, beaten, for brushing
Parmesan cheese, for sprinkling

Combine the oil, water, and salt. Then add the flour. Do not knead the dough. Mix just enough to combine the ingredients. If the dough is too soft, add a small amount of flour.

Preheat the oven to 375°.

To assemble the borekas, start with a ball of dough about the size of a golf ball. Roll to an oval shape. Add a heaping tablespoon of filling, then bring the top and bottom together, and seal the edges. This can be done with a tool, or by pinching and turning the open edge to make a fluted edge.

Brush the tops with the beaten egg and sprinkle with Parmesan cheese.

Bake on ungreased baking sheet for 20 to 30 minutes, until lightly browned.

TIPS & TRICKS:

- Borekas can be made and frozen to be cooked at a later time. This is accomplished by placing the formed borekas on a baking sheet and freezing. Place the frozen borekas in a lined box and return to the freezer until ready to use.

PUMPKIN BOREKAS

Esther Maimon

"My mother made this delightful pastry to be used at Rosh Hashanah as part of the service before the meal."

Makes about 45 borekas

Filling:
1 29-ounce can solid pumpkin, not pre-spiced
1 cup sugar
1 teaspoon cinnamon
1 egg, well-beaten
1/8 teaspoon ground cloves

Strain the pumpkin through a cheese cloth until no liquid remains, then combine with the sugar, cinnamon, egg, and cloves.

Dough:
1 cup oil
¾ cup sweet white wine
2 teaspoons sugar
2¾ to 3¾ cup flour

Cinnamon-sugar, for sprinkling

Mix the oil, wine, and sugar together. Slowly add the flour until the dough pulls away from the bowl. The dough gets oily as it sits; add a small amount of flour to each ball as needed.

Form the dough into small balls about 1 inch in diameter. Roll each ball out to about a 3-inch circle. Place a teaspoon of filling to the side of the center. Flip the dough over the filling to make a half-moon shape. Trim off excess dough on the ends as necessary. Seal the ends by fluting or by using a fork or other tool.

Preheat the oven to 375°.

Place the borekas on an ungreased baking sheet. Sprinkle the tops with a mixture of cinnamon and sugar. Bake for 15 minutes, until light golden-brown.

TIPS & TRICKS:

- Shortcut: Roll out some dough and use a cookie cutter (oval shape) to roll out several 3-inch circles at once.

BOYOS DE SPINACA

Madeline Caston Sherman

"Since the time of the expulsion of the Jews from Spain, during the Spanish Inquisition, Sephardic communities dispersed around the world and created recipes influenced by the culinary traditions of Morocco, Greece, Rhodes, Turkey, and India.

"Hospitality was a way of life in the early 20th century, as there were no televisions, Cineplexs, or computers, and people frequently visited each other without the need of an invitation. For these occasions, Turkish coffee, cookies, and homemade sweets were served. Sephardic kitchens were the place where sumptuous treats were labored over with love; a place where lively conversation mixed with the aroma of boyos baking. For celebrations, ladies from the Sephardic Bikur Cholim and Ezra Bessaroth in Seattle used to congregate at the synagogues to create an array of foods that smelled and tasted like none other!

"Before the advent of triple-washed spinach, grandmothers and daughters would wash and rinse the spinach several times to be certain it was clean. They would then chop the spinach and spread it over a cloth to dry overnight. Traditionally, boyos de spinaca are warmed and served with hard-boiled eggs, plain vanilla yogurt, and coffee at breakfast. Over the years, they have evolved as a favorite appetizer. They are considered a Sephardic delicacy, and I pass this recipe along in hopes of keeping alive a lost art of the Sephardic tradition."

Makes 3 or 4 dozen boyos

Dough:
1¼ teaspoon yeast (½ packet)
4 cups warm water
2 cups vegetable oil
Pinch of salt
8 to 10 cups flour

Filling:
40 ounces bagged spinach, triple washed
1 cup flour plus more, for dusting
2 cups feta cheese
3 cups Parmesan cheese, grated
1 cup vegetable oil
1 egg, beaten

Finely chop the washed spinach. Spread it out on a large cloth and let dry overnight.

Dissolve the yeast in the warm water, stirring to blend. Add the oil and salt. Slowly add the flour, stirring until the mixture starts to pull away from the bowl. Work the dough with your hands. The dough should not be sticky, rather pliable and easy to roll out. Cover the dough with a tea towel and let rise for about 1 hour.

To make the filling, place the spinach in a large mixing bowl and lightly dust with flour.

Mix the feta cheese, 2 cups of the Parmesan cheese, and the beaten egg and combine with the spinach.

Fill three small bowls: one with the remaining cup of the Parmesan cheese, another with the vegetable oil, and the last with 1 cup of flour.

Create dough patties by pinching enough of the dough to roll into a 4-inch ball. Place the dough patties on a rimmed baking sheet with ¼ inch of oil. Take one dough patty and stretch it out as thinly as possible, by hand, on a large board dusted with flour. You can use a rolling pin if you prefer.

Drizzle the dough with oil, sprinkle with Parmesan cheese, then cut the dough into two or three pieces. Place 1 tablespoon of the filling at one end and sprinkle with a pinch of flour. Roll the dough over the filling, tucking in the edges as you go. Dip in the Parmesan cheese and place on a rimmed baking pan with a ¼-inch of oil. Parchment paper can be used instead of the oil.

Preheat the oven to 400°.

Place the boyos on the lowest shelf of the oven for 20 to 30 minutes, until the pastries are browned on the bottom. Remove from the oven and cool on wire racks.

TIPS & TRICKS:

❖ If you want to freeze the boyos, place them on baking sheets in one layer. Place the baking sheet in the freezer until the boyos are frozen, then remove them and put them in a plastic bag until ready to reheat and enjoy.

"My Grandmother, Louise 'Kadune' Eskenazi, formerly Levy, came to Seattle by herself as a young teenager from Istanbul, Turkey. She was an outstanding baker, cook, and seamstress. Grama Kadune loved people and had a keen sense of humor. And, of course, her home was filled with delicious Sephardic foods."

~ Lynette Benaltabe

ONE-STEP CHEESE BOYICOS

Judith Amiel

"Traditionally, Sephardim eat a dairy lunch on Shabbat. This is one of the many cheese delicacies (e.g., borekas, bulemas, etc.) that are prepared on Friday for the family to enjoy the next day. These cheese boyicos are fast and easy to make, but most of all, a delicious treat.

"My mother made these frequently, and I have continued the tradition. I'm proud to say that my Ashkenazi-born daughter-in-law makes them for her family as well."

Makes about 40 boyicos

4 servings instant mashed potatoes or 4 baking potatoes, cooked and mashed
2½ cups flour
¾ cup oil
½ teaspoon baking soda
2 eggs, beaten
1 teaspoon salt
2 cups Parmesan cheese, grated and divided

Line a baking sheet with parchment paper and spray the paper with cooking spray.

Prepare the mashed potatoes and cool them slightly. Add the flour, oil, baking soda, eggs, salt, and 1⅔ cups of the Parmesan cheese, and mix very well with a spatula.

Preheat the oven to 375°.

To form the boyicos, take a generous tablespoonful of the mixture and form it into a ½-inch ball. Put the ball on the baking sheet. Press down softly on the ball with the back of a fork, making a pattern in the middle of the boyico. Do not flatten it completely. Repeat the process with the rest of the mixture.

Sprinkle the remaining Parmesan cheese over the boyicos. Bake for 20 to 25 minutes, until golden brown.

TIPS & TRICKS:

- Boyicos can be made larger, but make certain that you leave room between them so they do not stick together during baking.
- Boyicos can be frozen in zip-lock bags. They are great for aperitifs and hors d'oeuvres or just to enjoy as a special snack. To serve, thaw at room temperature and re-heat in a 250° oven for 15 minutes, until just heated through.

PAREVE POTATO KNISHES

Joani Diskin Saran

"In Spokane, every year we put on a dinner for 2500 people from the outside community. Many years ago, when I was chairman of this event, we decided to try some new side dishes to go with the brisket dinner. My beloved mother-in-law, Bert Diskin, and I created a recipe we called Potatoes Tzibella (potatoes with onions). Later we decided this would taste good as the filling for potato knishes. However, we weren't interested in kneading and stretching knish dough; that sounded like too much work to us. So we developed a recipe using puff pastry dough and instant potatoes. Amazingly, you can't tell they are instant potatoes. The trick to great knishes is in the pinching."

Makes 6 dozen large or 7½ dozen small knishes

1 box (15 to18 serving size) instant mashed potatoes (with no added salt)
1 10½-ounce can chicken-flavored stock
1 12-ounce package frozen chopped onions
1 cup margarine, melted and divided
Salt and white pepper, to taste
3 packages puff pastry sheets
Flour, for dusting
Oil

Make the instant potatoes according to package directions, except omit the margarine, substitute chicken flavored stock for the milk, and use slightly less water.

Sauté the frozen onions in ½ cup of the melted margarine until lightly brown. Add to potatoes. Add salt and pepper, to taste. The mixture should not be runny.

Open one sheet of puff pastry dough. Cut it into thirds along the folds. On a floured board, roll out one of the pieces to make it a slightly longer, thinner, and wider. Brush it with the remaining ½ cup of the margarine mixed with a little oil.

Place a mound of the potato mixture along the wide edge of the dough. Roll up, folding in the edges as you go. Leave the seam on the bottom side. Use the edge of your hand to cut and seal knishes. The desired size of the knishes will determine the number of cuts – 4 or 5 cuts will give you 5 or 6 nice-sized knishes. Each one will look like a little bed pillow. Carefully pinch and seal top and bottom corners. Tuck in corners of sealed edge to make a round knish with an indentation in the middle. At this point you can either bake or freeze the pastries. Repeat with the rest of the dough and the filling.

TIPS & TRICKS:

- The knishes can be frozen. Place the knishes on a waxed paper-lined baking sheet and place in the freezer. When the knishes are frozen, transfer to plastic bags and store in the freezer until ready to use. When ready to bake, follow the instructions above.

Preheat the oven to 400°.

Place the knishes in a buttered pan, leaving space between since they will puff up when they are baked. Bake for 30 to 45 minutes, until they are golden brown. These knishes are best when served warm.

PASSOVER KNISHES

Terry Bloom

Makes 18

Cooking spray
1 cup mashed potatoes (use your favorite recipe)
½ cup matzo meal
2 tablespoons potato starch, plus more for dusting
½ small yellow onion, finely diced
2 eggs, separated
½ teaspoon salt
½ teaspoon pepper
1 cup filling (see TIPS AND TRICKS)
½ cup poppy and/or sesame seeds, as a garnish

Preheat the oven to 350°. Spray a baking sheet with cooking spray.

Combine the mashed potatoes, matzo meal, potato starch, onion, egg whites, salt, and pepper. Knead the mixture to make a dough. Dust your hands and a pastry board with potato starch, and continue kneading the dough until it is no longer sticky.

Divide the dough into 18 balls, each about the size of a walnut. Flatten each ball to a small circle and put about a teaspoon of filling in the center. Close up the dough and make into a ball, sealing it well. Place the balls on the baking sheet.

Beat the reserved egg yolks and brush the egg wash on the tops of the balls. Sprinkle the balls with either poppy or sesame seeds, depending on your preference.

Bake the knishes for 25 to 35 minutes, until tops are golden brown. Serve hot.

TIPS & TRICKS:

- ❖ Use steamed broccoli, cheese, tapenade, or anything that sounds good to you for the filling. Just be sure to dice it finely.
- ❖ Depending on the filling, this dish can be pareve and vegetarian.

YAPRAKIES

Sharon Cordova Lott

"In the Sephardic culture, as in most cultures around the world, there is always time programmed for women chatting or, as we say in Ladino, 'Charlashon.' Today, we might call it coffee klatch, coffee or Starbucks time, or just meeting for a drink – of Diet Coke. Growing up, our 'Charlashon' revolved around Friday afternoon cooking, sampling, and lots of chatting. My mom, Frances Cordova, always used this time to sample her intricately homemade goodies and discuss everything that was going on in life with her sisters and friends. It was clear that all the women found satisfaction in sharing stories, experiences, and advice, as this was the group they trusted, admired, and whose opinions they appreciated most. My sister and I were always included in these Friday afternoon soirées, and we laughed and cried along with our mom, our aunts, and their friends. We felt the warmth and support of family and took pride in the Sephardic delicacies we helped create. We were delighted that it was our home in which all the women decided to congregate.

"Some days there may have been four or eight or ten women, but no matter how many people there were, every Friday around 4:00 p.m., everyone would cram around the kitchen table and drink coffee with plenty of cream and lots of sugar. Roscas (Ladino for rolls), boyos, yaprakies, and fila which might have been filled with spinach, potato, or pumpkin; biscochos, cheese, olives, fruit, and candy were typical of what appeared on our Friday afternoon table. Whatever the fare, with grape leaves fresh off the vine and perfect, fresh vegetables from my aunt's garden, the table resembled a still-life painting of one of the old masters. It was colorful, always adorned with glorious flowers, with food presented on gorgeous platters set on top of a beautiful lace tablecloth. My mother was the master of 'putting out a spread,' gathering women together, and making us all laugh. I revel in those memories, and I miss those days.

"From my mother, I learned much more than just the skill of hand-forming delicious Sephardic sweet and savory pastries. Perhaps the greatest lesson of all was about the value of making time for my women friends and appreciating their presence in my life. In our home today, I love the times our family and our friends – women and men alike –all spend in our kitchen, relishing in the joy of just being together, deepening our friendships, and creating memories for tomorrow."

2 tablespoons olive oil
3 onions, chopped
2 cups pearl rice
4 cups water, plus more for covering
Salt and pepper
1 tablespoon dried parsley
1 jar grape leaves
2 lemons, juiced

Heat the olive oil in a large fry pan and sauté the onions. Add the rice and 4 cups of the water and cook the rice according to the package directions. Season with salt and pepper. Add in the parsley and refrigerate until cool.

Preheat the oven to 350°.

TIPS & TRICKS:

- Uncooked yaprakies freeze very well.

Remove the grape leaves from the jar, unfold them, and snip the stems. Place a spoonful of the rice mixture into each grape leaf. Roll the leaf, envelope-style, and place in a single row in a 9x13-inch baking dish. Add the lemon juice and a touch of water to slightly cover the bottom of the dish. Season with a bit of pepper. Cover.

Bake for 30 minutes and serve hot or cold.

ARTICHOKE DIP

Tina Lippman Kahn

Serves 8

2 6-ounce jars artichoke hearts, drained and finely chopped
½ cup mayonnaise, adding more if desired
1 1½-ounce jar black caviar
5 eggs, hard-boiled and grated
¾ cup green onions, chopped

Blend the artichoke hearts with 1 tablespoon of the mayonnaise.

In a small clear glass bowl, layer the artichoke and mayonnaise mixture with the caviar, grated eggs, green onions, and a thin layer of mayonnaise. Repeat, then sprinkle with a few chopped green onions. Refrigerate until ready to serve. Use a small wooden serving spoon to serve. This is delicious with crackers of any kind.

TWO-TONED HUMMUS

Beth Fine

"This recipe combines my experiences while living in Israel in my twenties with my life in the Northwest for the last seventeen years. It begins with my basic hummus recipe, which I developed here in Seattle. The amounts of certain ingredients encourage you to taste as you go and decide how spicy/lemony/garlicky you are feeling on any given day. The roasted red pepper and chopped olive toppings go on top of the hummus to add some color and even more flavor. The whole dish can be made in a food processor."

Serves 8 to 10

Hummus:
1 can chick peas, drained and rinsed
1 to 2 lemons, juiced
2 to 4 cloves garlic, minced
¼ to ⅓ cup tahini
¼ to ⅓ cup water
2 to 4 tablespoons olive oil
1 teaspoons pepper
1 teaspoon cumin

Put the chick peas, juice of 1 lemon, 2 cloves garlic, ¼ cup of the tahini, ¼ cup of the water, 2 tablespoons of the olive oil, 1 tablespoon of the pepper, and the cumin in the food processor and blend for about two minutes, until silky. Taste and adjust seasonings to your liking, adding additional lemon juice, garlic, tahini, water, or olive oil for texture and taste.

Roasted Pepper Spread:
2 to 3 red peppers
½ lemon, juiced
1 to 2 cloves garlic
Several sprigs parsley

Lay the peppers on a baking sheet and place under a hot broiler. As the skin blisters, turn the peppers until they are soft and blistered on all sides. Remove from the oven, and let peppers rest for several minutes in a brown paper bag. Slip the skins off, core, and remove the seeds.

Put the red peppers, lemon juice, garlic, and parsley in the food processor and blend until you have a uniform texture. Adjust seasonings as you like.

Chopped Olive Spread:
1 cup pitted olives (black or kalamata olives)
1 to 2 cloves garlic
3 tablespoons pine nuts
2 tablespoons olive oil
½ lemon, juiced
Several sprigs parsley
1 tomato, diced (optional)
Black pepper to taste

Put the olives, garlic, pine nuts, olive oil, lemon juice, parsley, and tomato, if desired, in the food processor and blend until you have a uniform texture. Adjust seasoning as desired.

To assemble:
Spread the hummus across a shallow platter. Decorate with the red pepper and olive spreads; you can make one half red and the other black, a middle circle of red and outer circle of black, or whatever pleases your eye.

PEAR AND BLEU CHEESE CROSTINI

Carol Starin

"Growing up in the early 1950s, I never learned how to cook. I was usually assigned the salad – iceberg lettuce with a few vegetables. When I asked Mom how to make something, she frequently said, 'Oh, just throw in a can of mushroom soup.'

"As a young bride, I began taking cooking lessons – a lot of them. Some years ago, I took a week-long cooking course in Italy and ate in a wonderful trattoria in Sienna where crostini are a sign of hospitality. We experienced a fabulous crostini as a first course. I attempted to get the recipe from the waiter, but we had a communication problem. He didn't speak English and I didn't – and still don't – speak Italian. So this is my best guess. They are always a huge hit with company."

Makes 40 to 48 crostini

One baguette loaf approximately 22 to 24 inches long
1/3 cup olive oil
2 cloves garlic, halved
3/4 to 1 pound creamy bleu cheese
2 fresh pears, thinly sliced
1/4 to 1/3 cup honey

Slice the baguette on an angle into 40 to 48 pieces and toast on both sides. Brush the tops with olive oil and rub the cut garlic over the crostini.

Spread approximately 1 teaspoon of the bleu cheese on each piece of bread. Top the crostini with a thin slice of fresh pear, then drizzle with honey.

Just before serving, broil the crostini for one minute.

OVEN-ROASTED TOMATOES

Cindy Masin

"It was the aroma of these tomatoes roasting that caught my attention as I was about to savor this dish for the first time. The San Marzano tomatoes and the onions, sprinkled with a little bit of sugar, tend to caramelize during the four hours they are roasting. The tomatoes were served on a crostini spread with a thin layer of soft goat cheese and garnished with basil. Since then, I've come up with a few other ways to serve them: On pizza, with pasta, or the original way. This is one of the tastiest and most versatile dishes I have ever had."

Makes 20 to 24 tomatoes

½ cup extra virgin olive oil, divided
1 large sweet onion, finely chopped
2 cloves garlic, thinly sliced
1 tablespoon fresh rosemary, chopped
1 tablespoon fresh parsley, finely chopped
2 28-ounce cans whole peeled San Marzano tomatoes
1 heaping teaspoon sugar
Salt and pepper, to taste

Preheat the oven to 275°.

In a 9x13-inch glass dish, mix ¼ cup of the olive oil with the onion, garlic, rosemary, and parsley. Spread evenly over the bottom of the pan.

Drain the tomatoes and gently squeeze each one to release the juices, then place in a single layer over the onion mixture. Drizzle with the remaining ¼ cup of the olive oil. Sprinkle with the sugar, salt, and pepper to taste.

Bake the tomatoes for 4 hours and serve in a variety of ways.

TIPS & TRICKS:

- Use San Marzano tomatoes. They are available in many grocery stores or Italian specialty stores and are very sweet.
- Serving suggestions: As an appetizer, place a tomato on a crostini spread with goat cheese and garnished with fresh basil; on homemade pizza with fresh mozzarella cheese; or with pasta of any kind (i.e., with papparadelle noodles, garnished with freshly shaved Parmesan and chopped basil).

SPICY CHEESE CRACKERS

Darcy Goodman

"These crackers are wonderful all on their own just to snack on. But they also make a great accompaniment to any cold or hot soup or salad."

Makes 30 to 40 crackers

1 cup flour
¾ teaspoon salt
¼ teaspoon cayenne pepper
8 ounces sharp cheddar cheese, finely grated (about 2 cups)
½ cup butter, softened

In a bowl mix the flour, salt, and cayenne pepper. Add the cheddar cheese and butter. Working with your hands, blend the ingredients until a dough forms. Put the dough on a sheet of waxed paper and form into a log that is approximately 10-inches long and 1¼-inches in diameter. Roll the log in the wax paper and refrigerate for 2 hours.

Preheat the oven to 400°.

Slice the dough into ¼-inch thick rounds and arrange on an ungreased baking sheet about 1 inch apart. Bake for 16 to 18 minutes, until the edges are browned slightly. While hot, transfer the crackers to a rack until cool.

TIPS & TRICKS:

- If you prefer, the dough can be frozen after refrigeration then defrosted before cutting and baking.

EGGPLANT TOWER

Sarah Fishman

"This can easily be served as a vegetarian alternative or as a first course instead of salad. Not only does this dish taste delicious, its presentation is very impressive, served with a drizzle of balsamic syrup."

Serves 8

¾ cup balsamic vinegar
3 3-inch in diameter eggplants, sliced ½-inch thick
½ tablespoon olive oil, plus more for brushing
1 large sweet onion, sliced ⅓-inch thin, separated into onion rings
1 tablespoon butter
2 to 3 large balls fresh mozzarella, cut into ⅓-inch slices
4 large red peppers, halved lengthwise, seeded, and stem removed
¾ cup feta cheese, crumbled
16 large basil leaves, gently rinsed and dried on paper towels
16 medium oil-packed sun-dried tomatoes

In a small saucepan, heat the balsamic vinegar over medium heat for 10 to 15 minutes, stirring occasionally, until the vinegar is reduced by ⅓ and the syrup coats the back of a spoon. Cool.

Brush the eggplant slices with olive oil and grill until soft.

Melt the butter in a sauté pan over medium heat. Add ½ tablespoon of the olive oil and the onion slices. Sauté for 15 minutes, stirring often and allowing the onions to brown, but not burn, lowering the heat if necessary. Cover the pan and sweat the onions for 10 minutes over low heat. Uncover and continue sautéing until the onions are evenly browned and caramelized.

With a 3-inch cookie cutter, cut circles out of the red pepper pieces. Grill the red pepper pieces until slightly charred and pliable.

Preheat the oven to 375°.

Oil eight 3-inch ramekins. Layer as follows: Eggplant slice, 1 tablespoon of the caramelized onions, mozzarella, grilled pepper circle, 1 tablespoon of the feta cheese, 1 basil leaf, 1 sun-dried tomato, and top with another eggplant slice. Press into the ramekin. Repeat for each ramekin.

Bake the ramekins on a baking sheet for 20 minutes. Remove from the oven and let sit for 5 minutes. Run a knife around the edges to loosen, place a plate on top and flip to release. Decorate each plate with a smaller basil leaf and a sun-dried tomato. Drizzle with the balsamic syrup.

EGGPLANT DIP

Inez Caspi

"I came from a mixed family – a Sephardic mother and an Ashkenazi father – but the cooking in our home reflected the Sephardic roots. My Bulgarian grandmother, and later my mother, used to roast vegetables, especially peppers right in the fire on the burners of the stove. The tempting smell would permeate the house. A layer of black ash from the burning skins covered the stove and countertop and would drift into the air, landing on various surfaces in the kitchen. It took me few years to appreciate the value of roasting peppers in the oven. It was easier, cleaner, and maybe not as authentic, but the taste was almost as good. The following recipe combines some our favorite vegetables, roasted in the oven and then blended to create a wonderful dip. Eat with pita or pita chips."

Makes 3 cups

1 to 2 medium eggplants, peeled
2 red bell peppers, seeded and coarsely chopped
1 red onion, peeled and coarsely chopped
2 cloves garlic, minced
3 tablespoons olive oil
1½ teaspoon kosher salt
½ teaspoon black pepper

Preheat the oven to 400°.

In a large bowl, mix the eggplant, bell peppers, onion, garlic, olive oil, salt, and black pepper. Spread on a baking sheet and bake for 45 minutes.

Cool then blend in a food processor until smooth.

ARTICHOKE NIBBLES
Diane Cheifetz

"My special aunt, Sylvia Oseran, made this appetizer for many of her parties. She usually would cut them into one-bite squares, but, occasionally would serve them as a main dish to her mahjongg group, like a quiche with a salad."

Makes forty 2-inch square "nibbles" or 9 3x3-inch pieces

2 6-ounce jars marinated artichoke hearts
1 small onion, finely chopped
1 clove garlic, minced
4 eggs, beaten
1/4 cup bread crumbs
1/4 teaspoon salt
1/8 teaspoon pepper
1/8 teaspoon oregano
1/8 teaspoon Tabasco sauce
2 cups sharp cheddar cheese, shredded
2 tablespoons parsley, minced

Preheat the oven to 325°

Drain the marinade from one jar of the artichoke hearts into a medium size skillet. Drain the second jar, but discard the marinade. Chop the artichokes and set aside.

Heat the marinade in the skillet, add the onion and garlic, and sauté until the onion is limp, about 5 minutes.

Combine the eggs, bread crumbs, salt, pepper, oregano, and Tabasco sauce. Fold in the cheddar cheese and parsley. Add the artichokes and sautéed onion mixture, mixing well. Pour the mixture into an 8 or 9-inch square pan.

Bake for 30 minutes. Cool briefly, then cut into desired size.

TIPS & TRICKS:
- This appetizer can also be served cold.

APRICOT-GLAZED SALAMI

Todd Fishman

"This is sweet and tangy with a bit of heat and delicious for any holiday, football-watching party, or any other occasion you might want to serve it."

Serves 12 to 16

2 pounds whole kosher salami
1 14 to16-ounce jar apricot preserves
1 teaspoon dry mustard
1 tablespoon yellow mustard
Party rye bread
Honey mustard

Preheat the oven to 350°.

Slice the salami, but not all the way through, and place in a greased glass dish.

Mix the apricot preserves, dry mustard, and yellow mustard together and pour over the salami.

Bake for 70 minutes, basting every 20 minutes. The salami will have a glazed appearance and will be crispy around the edges. Serve with thinly-sliced party rye bread and honey mustard.

BLACK BEAN, CORN, AND RED ONION QUESADILLA

Doreen Alhadeff

"This is one of our favorites. It is best served on a separate plate with a slightly spicy pico de gallo, a bit of chopped avocado, and a dollop of sour cream. You will love it as an appetizer or starter course."

Serves 12

1 15-ounce can black beans, drained, rinsed, and patted dry
2 cups fresh, sweet white corn (3 to 4 ears), cut off the cob
1 cup red onion, finely chopped
2 cups Monterey jack cheese, shredded
2 cups extra sharp white cheddar cheese, shredded
12 tortillas
1 tablespoon oil
1 teaspoon cayenne pepper
Salsa, as a garnish
Avocado, chopped, as a garnish
Sour cream, as a garnish

Preheat the oven to 450°.

Toss the beans, corn, and red onions together. In a separate bowl, mix the Monterey jack and cheddar cheeses.

Place a piece of foil on a baking sheet. Spray it with nonstick spray.

Put 1 tortilla on the foil. Spoon 1/3 cup of the bean mixture over the tortilla. Sprinkle with 1/3 cup of the cheese mixture. Place the next tortilla on top and press down gently. Repeat with bean and cheese mixtures. Top with another tortilla and press down gently. Brush the top with a little oil and lightly sprinkle with cayenne pepper. Follow the same process with the next "stack."

Bake for 12 to 15 minutes, until golden brown. Cut into desired size wedges and serve on appetizer plates with really good salsa, avocado, and sour cream.

COWBOY SALSA

Andrea Lott

"My mom, sisters, and I have been making this recipe for years, and it is always a hit with everyone. It can be served with tortilla chips as an easy, fabulous, crowd-pleasing appetizer."

Makes 7 cups of salsa

1 15-ounce can whole kernel corn, drained
1 15-ounce can black beans, drained
1 15-ounce can black-eyed peas, drained
2 3.8-ounce cans sliced black olives, drained
5 medium tomatoes, chopped
2 jalapeños, finely chopped (more if you prefer a spicier salsa)
¾ bunch green onions, chopped
¼ cup red wine vinegar
¼ cup olive oil
Salt
3 to 4 large avocados, peeled and chopped

Mix the corn, black beans, black eyed peas, olives, tomatoes, jalapeños, and green onions together in a very large mixing bowl. Season with the red wine vinegar, olive oil, and salt. Mix, taste, and adjust seasoning if necessary. Just before serving, add the avocado and gently mix.

DEL'S CHICKEN DRUMETTES
Del Baron

Serves 8

1/3 cup soy sauce
1/3 cup sherry wine
1/3 cup water
1/4 cup brown sugar
1/2 teaspoon powdered ginger
2 to 4 green onions, sliced
1 pound chicken drumettes
Sesame seeds, as a garnish and for dipping
Sweet-hot mustard, for dipping

Preheat the oven to 350°. Grease a baking dish or pan.

Mix the soy sauce, sherry, water, sugar, ginger, and onions in a sauté pan and heat.

Place the drumettes on the prepared dish, pour the sauce over top, and cover with foil.

Bake for 1 hour. Remove the foil and bake until the liquid is absorbed. Sprinkle with sesame seeds and serve with sweet-hot mustard and sesame seeds on a bed of lettuce.

MOJITOS FOR A CROWD

Darcy Goodman

Serves 16

2 cups mint leaves, plus extra for garnishing
$1\frac{1}{3}$ cups fresh lime juice
$1\frac{1}{2}$ cups sugar
4 cups light rum
8 cups club soda

In a bowl, mash the mint, lime juice, and sugar. Let it sit for at least 15 minutes or up to 2 hours. Add the rum.

In a tall glass filled with ice, pour 3 tablespoons of club soda then enough rum mixture to top off the glass. Stir and garnish with a fresh mint sprig and serve.

TIPS & TRICKS:

- I usually sieve out the crushed mint before adding the rum.
- Homegrown mint is the best for this.
- Be sure the club soda is fresh and unopened.

MARGARITAS

Cindy Masin

Serves 10 to 12

"Easy and refreshing."

1 12-ounce can frozen limeade, thawed slightly
8 ounces Tequila
4 ounces triple sec
1 lime, juiced and 1 lime, sliced, as a garnish
2 to 3 cups ice, or more

Blend the limeade, tequila, triple sec, lime juice, and ice in a blender until smooth and slushy. Pour into a pitcher and place the pitcher in the freezer until ready to use. Stir and pour. Garnish with a slice of lime.

TIPS & TRICKS:

- For easy measuring of the tequila and triple sec, use the limeade can. Fill it $\frac{2}{3}$ full for the tequila and $\frac{1}{3}$ full for the triple sec.

TOM AND JERRYS

Marleen Magnoni Alhadeff

"This recipe was given to me by my mother, Lanore Manuel. She shared this wonderful and festive libation every New Year's Eve with the entire family and all the employees at the Italian restaurant owned by our family, who were the first to bring pizza to Walla Walla. Even though the restaurant closed some years ago, we continue the tradition at our home every New Year's Eve. It can be served to underage kids or non-drinkers without alcohol or with alcohol to those who prefer it."

Serves 16 to 20

1 pound butter
2 pounds powdered sugar
12 eggs, separated
1 teaspoon cinnamon
½ teaspoon ground cloves
½ teaspoon allspice
½ teaspoon nutmeg
Hot water
Whiskey and brandy (optional)

Beat the butter and sugar until creamy.

In another bowl, beat the egg yolks with a fork until creamy, then add to the butter mixture.

Beat the egg whites until soft peaks form and blend into the butter mixture. Add the cinnamon, cloves, allspice, and nutmeg. Refrigerate the batter if it is not to be used immediately.

To serve, spoon 1 tablespoon of batter into a mug and add hot water for a non-alcoholic beverage. For a spirited drink, follow the same process as above but leave room to add one-half jigger of whiskey and one-half jigger of rum or brandy.

TIPS & TRICKS:

❖ Batter can be made same day or night before event, but be sure to refrigerate when not using; it can be frozen or kept in refrigerator for several weeks.

Like Challah from Heaven

"It is impossible to talk about traditions in Jewish cooking without mentioning bagels," writes Cindy Masin.

Cindy is right. Although the origin of the bagel is unknown, we do know that the *bajgiel* was a mainstay in Polish Jewish cookery by the end of the 16th century. The round shape lent itself to circle-of-life celebrations like circumcision meals and shiva calls; the hole in the middle gave it existential significance ("Now you have a mere zero," mused Yiddish writer Eliezar Shteynberg); its favoritism led Murray Lender of Lender's Bagels to call it "a Jewish English muffin with personality." The bagel has influenced both Ashkenazi Jewish mealtime customs and left an indelible stamp on American Jewish culture. Interestingly, while the bagel's popularity exploded in America, it barely made a ripple in Israel, where the cuisine went down another track.

Although New York has unofficially claimed the bagel as its state food, bagels and breads are integral to Washington State Jewish history, too. Arlene Mosler Schuster pays tribute here to her grandfather, Sam Mosler, who opened the New York Bakery on Jackson Street in Seattle in 1899. Jerry Cone's bagels, a project he sweetly shares now with his grandson, were inspired by his visits to Brenner Brothers Bakery throughout his young life until the beloved bakery moved. Our bagel recipe submitters have spent years developing the "perfect" bagel out here in inferior bagel territory.

As much as bagels are central to the Jewish-American table, no bread is more Jewishly significant than challah. The two braided loaves on the Shabbat table signify the double portion of manna that the Israelites received in the desert on Shabbat. Leviticus (24:5–6) commanded the Israelites to place 12 loaves of challah on the table before God in the tent of meeting on Shabbat. This holy table symbolically evolved into the Shabbat table, and mealtime, especially on Shabbat, is considered a holy rite among religious families. "Taking challah," the ritual of setting aside a small piece of the dough for the Kohen (ancient priest), has been done throughout history and is one of the three mitzvot central to women. While the braids are imbued with symbolism, this is more likely a development; challah does not need to be braided, and in fact Sephardic and Mizrachi Jews have historically used entirely different breads for challah. Furthermore, many challah bakers have taken liberties to shape challah into other meaningful, or just fun, designs and to doctor them up with sweet and savory flavors.

TIDBIT:

To "get bageled" can mean many things, but around 2007 the term was coined to refer to Jews who make themselves known to other Jews, usually by making cryptic Jewish cultural references. If anyone has ever made an offhand remark about, say, blintzes in your general direction and followed up with a nod or a conversation about Jewish identity, you've been bageled.

Jessica Levine Kupferberg. "Have You Ever Been Bageled?" *www.jweekly.com.*

Challah recipes generally call for similar ingredients, but the bread invites innovation. Leah Jaffee suggests adding the various flours symbolic of the Holy Land and changing out refined sweeteners for natural ones, and Gilah Kletenik shares her recipe for wheat-free challah made with spelt flour. At the same time, challah stands for an age-old practice lovingly handed down from one generation to the next. Karen Hudesman reflects on her children, who, as little ones, braided their own challot with their tiny hands, reminding her Polish immigrant parents of the old country.

"Challah." *Wikipedia.*
Glenn C. Altschuler. "Three Centuries of Bagels." *The Jewish Daily Forward.*
Claudia Roden. "Challah." *MyJewishLearning.com.*
"The History of Challah." *Nycookery.blogspot.com.*

LIKE CHALLAH FROM HEAVEN

TRIED AND TRUE CHALLAH

Karen Hudesman

"Baking is my passion, so here is one of my favorite recipes. I have made this Challah since my kids were small, all gathered in the kitchen with their tiny little hands in the flour, rolling the dough, braiding it and making their own individual challahs. All the family dinners were at our home, and a holiday was not complete without our famous challah. Both of my parents were immigrants from Poland, and when I would bake this challah and Biscotti (page 226) it reminded them of the 'Old Country'."

Makes 2 loaves

Sponge:
3 tablespoons active dry yeast
3 cups warm water
½ cup sugar
3 cups flour

Dough:
4 teaspoons salt
¾ cup canola oil
½ cup sugar
4 eggs
6 to 8 cups flour

Egg Wash:
1 egg
2 tablespoons milk

Poppy seeds or sesame seeds, as a garnish

Mix the yeast with warm water, sugar, and flour on low speed until the mixture is smooth, about 2 to 3 minutes. Let the sponge rise 30 to 40 minutes or until it doubles in size.

For the dough, add the salt, oil, sugar, and eggs to the sponge. Slowly add enough of the 6 to 8 cups of flour to make a silky, satin dough. Knead the dough until it is the texture of your skin, and then place the dough in a greased bowl.

Cover the bowl with a towel and let the dough rise in a warm spot until it doubles in size. Punch the dough down and divide it into 2 portions.

Divide each portion into 3 parts. Roll each part into a long rope. Braid 3 ropes into a loaf, and repeat with the other 3 ropes, making 2 loaves. Let the loaves rest for 45 minutes.

Preheat the oven to 350°. Put the loaves on a lightly greased baking sheet. Beat the remaining egg with the milk and brush the wash onto the loaves. Sprinkle the loaves with poppy seeds or sesame seeds.

Bake for 35 to 45 minutes. Loaves will be golden brown when done, and the dough between the pieces of the braid will not look wet or gooey.

TU B'SHEVAT WHOLE WHEAT CHALLAH

Leah Jaffe

"This recipe for whole wheat challah is sweetened with honey and barley malt syrup (available in the organic section) without any refined white sugar. I've also added a little oat bran. I didn't have any rye flour or spelt flour, or I would have thrown some in to complete the grains of the Holy Land. If you have some at home, substitute some of the wheat flour for the others. This challah has a wonderful crumb and a deep richness, and, of course, it is great throughout the year shaped into sandwich loaves.

"The ratio of whole wheat to white flour is 3:2, so the loaf is still on the lighter side. If you regularly eat the classic egg challah, consider changing it up a bit with this tasty whole wheat option. I've used the six-braid for these loaves, representing the twelve tribes of Israel."

Makes 4 loaves

2 cups oat bran
9 cups whole wheat flour
7 cups unbleached white flour
6 packages active dry yeast
3 tablespoons salt
¾ cup honey
¼ cup barley malt syrup
5 eggs
4 cups lukewarm water
1 cup oil

Combine the oat bran, both types of flours, yeast, and salt in a large mixing bowl and give it a quick whisk to blend.

Combine the honey, malt syrup, eggs, water, and oil in a medium bowl. Add the wet ingredients to the flour mixture.

If using a mixer with a dough hook, blend at a low speed for 2 minutes. Increase the speed slightly and beat for an additional 2 minutes. Reduce the speed to low and knead for 12 minutes. If mixing by hand, mix until combined. Turn out to work surface and knead for 12 minutes. The dough should be neither sticky nor stiff.

Shape the dough into a ball. Lightly oil a large bowl and put the ball into the bowl upside down. Use it to smear the oil around the bowl and then bring it right side up. Cover the bowl with a dish towel and set aside to rise until doubled in bulk, about 1 hour.

Once the dough has risen, punch down and move it to the work table. Divide the dough into quarters and shape into balls. Cover and let rest for 30 minutes.

Cut each ball into the number of strands you'd like to braid to form each loaf (I use 6 strands for this challah). After braiding, move the challah to a baking sheet. Brush with a beaten egg and set aside, uncovered, to rise until almost doubled in bulk. Depending on the temperature in the room, this could be up to another hour.

Preheat the oven to 350°. Bake the challah for about 25 to 30 minutes, until golden brown. The loaves should sound hollow when patted on the bottom.

TIPS & TRICKS:

❖ To see a video of how to make this challah, go to www.LeahCooksKosher.com.

SPELT CHALLAH

Gilah Kletenik

Makes two 8½x4½-inch loaves

1 tablespoon active dry yeast
2 cups water (105 to 110°)
3 tablespoons honey
3 tablespoons butter, melted
2 teaspoons sea salt
6 cups spelt flour (use any combination of whole or white spelt)

Combine the yeast, water, and honey in a large warm bowl. Let it stand for 10 minutes or until the yeast softens.

Stir in the butter, salt, and 3 cups of the flour. Stir vigorously with a wooden spoon. Add the remaining flour in small quantities until the dough becomes too stiff to stir. Place the dough on lightly floured surface.

Knead for about 6 minutes, adding any remaining flour as necessary, until the dough becomes smooth and elastic. Do not over-knead.

Place the dough in a lightly greased bowl. Cover and let rise in a warm, draft-free spot for about 2 hours or until doubled in bulk.

Grease two 8½x4½-inch loaf pans.

Punch down the dough to deflate it and divide it in half. Form each half into a smooth loaf and place in a prepared pan.

Cover and let rise in a warm, draft-free spot for about 1 hour or until the dough rises to the top of the pans.

Preheat the oven to 350°. Uncover the risen loaves. Place the pans on a heavy baking sheet and bake for 45 minutes or until the tops are light brown and crusty. Remove from the oven and tap out of the pan onto the baking sheet.

Turn the oven off and return the breads to the oven to crisp for 5 additional minutes. Remove from the oven and let cool on a wire rack.

TIPS & TRICKS:

- For a lighter flavor and texture, use up to 50% white spelt flour.
- It is possible to add fresh thyme, garlic, kalamata olives, sautéed onions, or any other fresh herbs or ingredients of this kind to the dough before baking.
- For an even sweeter bread, sprinkle the dough lightly with cinnamon sugar and gently roll it into the dough before rising.

"Mildred Rosenbaum, a co-founder of Washington State Jewish Historical Society (WSJHS) and my mother, always tells me she uses a challah recipe, given to her by Jeanette Schrieber, the other co-founder of WSJHS. I have since learned that she incorporates elements from a recipe by Risha Dadoun, the daughter of her dear friend Stella Bay.

"My mother always baked challot on Shabbat, recalling that her own mother, a rebbetsin on the American prairie, did so while raising six children. She never liked her mother's recipes but loved Jeannette's – and Risha's!

"Mother, who was burned badly in childhood, rarely used her hands except to make her challah. I still see her standing over the dough, but I prefer to use an electric mixer."

~ Betsy Schneier

JERRY CONE'S BAGELS

Jerry Cone

"Going to Brenner's on Cherry Street for freshly baked bagels began for me when I was a kid and continued on into married life until Brenner Brothers Bakery moved. That was long before bagels could be found in every grocery store. And that's when I started to create, boil, and bake those little holes with dough around them. When my grandson, Sam, wanted his 'great papa' to let him help, I joyfully complied."

Makes 12 bagels

1 package active dry yeast
1½ teaspoons kosher salt
3 cups all-purpose unbleached flour
⅔ cups lukewarm water
2 tablespoons sugar
3 tablespoons vegetable oil
1 egg

Egg Wash (optional):
1 egg white
1 tablespoon water
Poppy seeds or sesame seeds

In an electric mixer, combine yeast and salt with 1 cup of the flour. Stir in lukewarm water and sugar. Add the oil and the egg. Beat until very smooth. Add the remaining flour, ½ cup at a time, to make a soft dough.

Move the dough to a lightly-floured surface. Knead a minute or two until dough is smooth and elastic. Place the dough into a lightly-oiled bowl. Cover with a dish towel and let the dough rise at room temperature for about 1 hour or until doubled in bulk.

Punch down and transfer the dough to a lightly floured surface. Knead briefly. Divide the dough into 12 equal pieces. Roll each piece into a log, about 6 inches long and ¾-inch thick, and pinch the ends together to make a circle. Place the bagels back on the floured surface and cover with a towel. Let rise 45 minutes.

Preheat the oven to 375°. Bring 4-quarts of water to a gentle boil in a large pot. Slide each bagel into the water. After 30 seconds, flip them over and simmer for 3 minutes. Remove from the water with a large slotted spoon or spatula and drain on paper towels.

Once the bagels have drained, place them on a lightly-oiled baking sheet. If preferred, you can brush the bagels with an egg wash and add toppings. Mix the egg white and water and then sprinkle the bagels with sesame or poppy seeds.

Bake at 375° for 10 minutes then increase the temperature to 400° and bake for an additional 10 to 15 minutes, until golden brown.

ONE-HOUR CHEWY BAGELS

Mike Cheifetz

"I wanted a chewy bagel, with a substantial crust, and just basic good bread flavor. I could not find a bagel recipe that met all of my specifications, so I decided to create my own. At first, the process took longer than I hoped and required more clean up than I wanted. And so, I have now developed a recipe and procedures that meet my expectations. I find that weighing the ingredients, like the flour, results in the most accurate measurements. But I have approximated the flour measurements into cups for convenience in this recipe. This should take you just over an hour, and leave you a bowl, a cooling rack, and 2 spoons to wash, and a bread board to quickly scrape or brush off."

Makes 8 bagels

3⅓ cups (450 grams) unbleached white bread flour
⅔ cup (90 grams) gluten flour
1 tablespoon sugar
1½ teaspoons salt
2 packages active dry yeast
1 tablespoon oil
1½ cups water, heated in the microwave on high for 1 minute
1 teaspoon baking powder

Add the flours, sugar, salt, yeast, and oil into the bowl of an electric mixer fitted with a dough hook. Drizzle the heated water down the side of bowl while the mixer is on low, and watch until the flour is completely incorporated. Usually, there will be a small quantity of water left, but all the water may be required. Don t use more water.

Set a timer for 7 minutes, and let the mixer knead the dough on medium speed. When the dough "climbs the hook," turn up the mixer speed a notch. If some of the dough creates a separate "baby," you can stop the mixer, pull the dough off the hook, re-form a ball, lower the hook into the ball, and start the mixer again. When the knead time is up, pull the dough off the hook, form it into a smooth ball, and drop it back into the mixer bowl and cover with a towel. There should be no need to oil the bowl if you have measured carefully. Allow the dough to rise for 10 minutes.

Preheat the oven to 420°.

Wet a pizza stone, or equivalent, and place on bottom rack of the oven. When the dough has risen sufficiently, drop it onto a bread board (there should be no need to flour the board if you have measured carefully), and roll into a log about 16 inches long. The dough will be springy. You will need to stretch the dough then let it spring back to the size you want.

Divide the dough into 8 pieces. Roll each piece into a snake. Form the snake into a bagel by placing the ends together over your hand and roll beneath your palm until the seam is joined. Set all the bagels aside.

In a very large pot, bring 10 cups water and the baking soda to a boil. Drop the bagels into the bath one at a time. If they sink, wait until they surface, and then boil each bagel for 15 seconds, flip, and boil another 15 seconds. Remove the bagels to a wire rack (use a towel, if you must, but some dough will stick).

Place the bagels on a baking sheet lined with parchment paper. Place the baking sheet on the hot rack above the pizza stone for 12 minutes, flip the bagels and bake another 12 minutes.

Let the bagels cool and enjoy them while they are fresh!

TIPS & TRICKS:

- ❖ If you want all the above results, you will need a mixer with a bread hook, a scale, and a pizza stone or equivalent.
- ❖ To get the chewy texture, I add gluten flour to my recipe. Try Bob's Red Mill brand.
- ❖ If you do not have an electric mixer with a dough hook, this recipe is not for you. You can find others that assume you will knead the dough by hand.
- ❖ Skip the scale at your own peril. If you follow closely by weight, you will not need to flour your bread board, and will have minimal cleanup.
- ❖ The pizza stone is not an absolute (you can instead use a terra-cotta planter drip pan) or you can toss boiling water in a preheated pan in the oven when you load the bagels in the oven, but if you skip the steam, you will not get as good a crust. The trick with the stone is that it will absorb water, and when the oven heats, provide steam.
- ❖ I make 8 bagels with the quantities listed above. To make more or fewer bagels, divide the dough into the desired number of pieces. I designed this to exactly fit our small oven and pans.

BAGELS

Cindy Masin

"I found the recipe for these bagels in an old cookbook, The Breads of France *(published in 1976). On our first trip to Paris in 1985, we stopped in at Jo Goldenberg's Deli in the Marais because I just had to see for myself the place where the absolute best crispy-on-the-outside-and-chewy-in-the-middle bagel I had ever tasted was first baked. For a while, being busy with kids and so many other activities, I made them only occasionally, but knowing of this cookbook project, I was positive this is a recipe people would love to make and their families would love to eat. Besides, it is impossible to talk about traditions in Jewish cooking without mentioning bagels."*

Makes eight 4 to 5-inch bagels or twelve 3-inch bagels

¼ cup yellow cornmeal
1½ cups lukewarm water
2 packages dry yeast
1 tablespoon salt
4 tablespoons sugar, divided
3 to 4 cups all-purpose flour, approximately

Egg Wash:
1 egg white
1 tablespoon water

Sesame seeds, kosher salt, poppy seeds, or onion bits, for sprinkling (optional)

Prepare a baking sheet by fitting it with a piece of parchment paper, thoroughly greasing it, and sprinkling it with the cornmeal.

Pour the water and yeast into the bowl of an electric mixer. Stir to dissolve and leave for 3 to 4 minutes until yeast is creamy. Stir in the salt and 3 tablespoons of the sugar. Add 2 cups of the flour and beat at low speed for 1 minute, then turn to high for 3 minutes. Return mixer to low speed and add 1 more cup of the flour, mixing until incorporated.

Place the dough under a dough hook for 4 to 5 minutes. If the dough sticks to the side of the bowl, add additional flour, one tablespoon at a time, as necessary. Bagel dough must be firm, so add enough flour to make it solid when pinched with fingers. If kneading by hand, do so with strong push-turn-fold rhythm. If the dough is still sticky or elastic, add flour.

When it is ready, place the dough in a clean and greased bowl. Cover it tightly with plastic wrap and leave it undisturbed at room temperature until doubled in volume.

While the dough is rising, bring 2 quarts of water to a boil and add the remaining tablespoon of sugar. Reduce the heat and keep the water simmering.

To shape the bagels, turn the dough out onto a flour-dusted work surface and punch down. Divide the dough into 8 or 12 pieces depending on the desired bagel size. Shape each piece into a ball. Allow the dough to sit for 3 or 4 minutes before flattening each piece with the palm of your hand. With your thumb, press deep into the center of the bagel to tear it open. Pull the hole open and smooth the rough edges with the fingers. Repeat until all bagels are formed. Leave the bagels on the work surface, covered with waxed paper, for about 10 minutes.

Preheat the oven to 450°.

With the water simmering, lift 1 bagel at a time and lower it into the water. It should sink then rise to the top. Only do 2 or 3 at a time, since the bagels will expand slightly. Let the bagels sit for 25 seconds, flip them, and let them sit for another 25 seconds. Lift bagels out with a skimmer, drain briefly on a towel, then place on the prepared baking sheet. As the bagels come out of the water, they will be shiny, thanks to the sugar.

With a fork, beat the egg white and water for the egg wash. Brush the top of the bagels with the glaze, then sprinkle with your choice of topping or, if you wish, leave the bagels plain.

Put the bagels on the middle shelf of the oven to bake for 35 minutes total. About 17 minutes through the baking, turn the bagels over. This will keep them in a rounded shape. Remove from the oven when brown and shiny, and place them on a rack to cool.

TIPS & TRICKS:

- You can add 1 cup of whole wheat flour to replace a cup of all-purpose flour.
- Try making cinnamon raisin bagels by adding a teaspoon of cinnamon and ½ cup raisins to the dough.
- Bagels can be made smaller if you prefer.
- It is possible to make the dough, put it in a greased bowl covered with plastic wrap, and refrigerate it until the next morning. The dough will double in size in the refrigerator. To proceed, remove the dough from the refrigerator and let the dough sit for 30 minutes before following the above steps to form and bake the bagels.

HOMEMADE MATZO (UNLEAVENED BREAD)

Miriam Coates

"'This is the bread of affliction,' my father would drone every Passover as he opened the familiar blue square box. 'Matzo is tasteless and dry, not meant to be enjoyed. Eating it should remind you of the sufferings of our people.' As he went on and on and on with his yearly lecture on the harshness of slavery and unleavened bread, I sat there slathering on salted butter and devouring sheet after sheet of crispy goodness. Although bland and stomach-binding, this so-called 'bread of affliction' was a welcome change to the squishy, faintly chemical-smelling Wonder Bread loaves my mother bought the rest of the year. Despite the family mandate that matzo eating required a certain degree of complaining to make it religiously significant, my appreciation for the magical combination of flour, water, and fire was born.

"When I grew up in the Midwest during the 1970s there were only two kinds of matzo available, Manischewitz and Streit's. Both perfectly square and almost identical in taste, matzo was matzo....or so I thought. It was not until decades later at a community Seder that I discovered that matzo could be round, organic, or made from non-white flour. Gourmet matzo? Forget the family mandate. My quest for the ultimate 'bread of affliction' was ignited. After sampling every brand and flavor of matzo I could find, it hit me. My ancestors did not eat matzo found on supermarket shelves. They made it. By hand. And you can too! Affliction never tasted so good."

Makes two 6x6-inch sheets

2 cups flour (not self-rising)
1 cup water
Kosher salt (optional)

Preheat the oven with a baking stone or cooking sheet to 475°.

Mix the flour and water. Knead until the mixture forms a non-sticky dough, adding more flour if necessary. Roll into thin sheets using either a rolling pin or a pasta machine set to 4. Cut the sheets of rolled dough into rectangles or squares with a pasta cutter or straight edged knife. Prick the surface of the dough evenly with a fork. Sprinkle with salt if desired.

Slide the sheets of dough onto the baking stone and bake for 4 minutes or until matzo is slightly browned. Remove the matzo from the oven and cool on a wire rack.

DILLY CASSEROLE BREAD

Goldie Silverman

"This is the only bread I know how to make. It was the winner of the Pillsbury Bake-Off Contest in 1960, and I have been baking it ever since. My father loved it and even though my mother and I had the same recipe, he swore it was better when I made it."

Makes 2 loaves

5 cups flour, divided
4 tablespoons sugar
4 tablespoons instant minced onions
4 teaspoons dill seed
2 teaspoons salt
½ teaspoon baking soda
2 packages active dry yeast
½ cup water
2 tablespoons margarine or butter, room temperature
2 cups small curd cottage cheese
2 eggs
4 teaspoons margarine or butter, melted
½ teaspoon salt if desired

In a large bowl, combine 2 cups of the flour, sugar, onion, dill, salt, baking soda, and yeast. Mix well.

In a small saucepan, heat the water, 2 tablespoons of the margarine or butter, and the cottage cheese until very warm (120° to 130°). Add warm mixture and eggs to the flour mixture. Blend at low speed until moistened. Beat for an additional 3 minutes at medium speed.

By hand, stir in the remaining 3 cups of flour to form a stiff batter. Cover loosely with greased plastic wrap and cloth towel. Let rise in a warm place (80° to 85°) until light and doubled in size, about 45 to 60 minutes.

Generously grease two 1½ to 2-quart casseroles. Punch the dough to remove all the air bubbles then divide the dough between the two casseroles. Cover, then let the dough rise again in a warm place until light and doubled in size, 30 to 40 minutes.

Preheat the oven to 350°. Uncover the dough and bake the bread 30 to 40 minutes or until loaf is dark golden brown and sounds hollow when lightly tapped. If necessary, cover with foil to prevent over-browning. Let the bread stand for 10 minutes, then remove from the casserole and place on a wire rack. Brush with the melted margarine or butter and sprinkle with salt. Cool for 15 minutes. Serve warm or cool.

HEARTY WHOLE WHEAT BREAD

Arlene Mosler Schuster

"This recipe is based on a bread concocted by my father, George Mosler, who came from a family of professional bakers and baked extensively as a hobby. It is so delicious that, years after tasting my father's bread, I was able to recreate it, and my family agrees that it has the same taste and hearty, nutritional appeal. My grandfather, Sam Mosler, opened the New York Bakery at 600 Jackson Street in Seattle in 1899. A baker, originally from Austria, Sam moved to Seattle five years after coming to the United States."

Makes two 9x5-inch loaves

3 cups whole wheat flour
3 to 4 cups unbleached, all-purpose flour, divided
⅓ cup light brown sugar
1 teaspoon salt
2 packages rapid rise yeast
1½ teaspoons Cook's Vanilla Powder
¼ cup flax seed
¼ cup wheat germ
¼ cup honey
¼ cup canned pumpkin
1 cup half-and-half, lukewarm
1 cup warm water (warmed to 110°)
6 tablespoons butter, melted, plus more for brushing
1 egg, beaten

Stir together in a large bowl the whole wheat flour, 2 cups of the all-purpose flour, brown sugar, salt, yeast, vanilla powder, flax seed, and wheat germ.

Add the honey, pumpkin, half-and-half, water, butter, and egg. Combine thoroughly, adding enough all-purpose flour so that the dough can be turned out onto a floured board.

Knead the dough for 8 to 10 minutes, adding more flour as necessary to keep the mixture from sticking to the board. The dough will remain slightly tacky due to the honey. Place the dough in a lightly greased bowl, cover with a towel, and allow the dough to rise until it doubles in bulk, about 1½ hours.

Punch down the dough and let rise again for 30 minutes.

Grease two 9x5-inch loaf pans. Divide the dough into two equal parts, then round up each piece of dough and let it rest 5 minutes more.

Form the loaves by shaping each dough part into a rectangle. Fold each side of the rectangle to the approximate size of the loaf pan. Roll it slightly to form a tight cylinder.

Compress each loaf, seam side down, into the lightly greased pans. Cover and let rise 45 minutes more in the loaf pans.

TIPS & TRICKS:

- ❖ Cooks Vanilla Powder is the secret ingredient to this fabulous-tasting bread.
- ❖ Freeze the remaining canned pumpkin in ¼ cup portions to use the next time you bake the bread.
- ❖ Using non-stick pans will shorten the baking time

Preheat the oven to 350°. Bake for 30 to 40 minutes, until the loaves sound hollow when tapped on the bottom or an instant read thermometer measures 190°.

Remove the loaves from the pans and place onto a cooling rack. Brush with the melted butter or margarine.

MOLASSES OATMEAL BREAD

Marcie Stone

"Here's a bread that I make and love – it is hearty, somewhat sweet, and rather dense. It makes great toast!"

Makes 2 loaves

2 packages active dry yeast
½ cup lukewarm water
5 to 6 cups flour, sifted and divided
2 cups uncooked old-fashioned oats
1 teaspoon salt
1 cup water
½ cup milk
½ cup molasses
½ cup margarine
2 eggs, at room temperature

Dissolve the yeast in the lukewarm water. In a large bowl of an electric mixer, combine 1 cup of the flour with the oats and salt. In a saucepan over low heat, combine the 1 cup water, milk, molasses, and margarine. Heat until the liquids are warm to the touch – not hot. Remove from the heat, then add the yeast mixture.

Gradually add the liquid mixture to the dry ingredients and beat for 2 minutes at medium speed. Add the eggs and ¾ cup of the flour (or enough to make a thick batter) and beat at high speed for 2 minutes. Continue adding flour to make the dough soft. Turn the dough out onto a lightly floured board and knead until smooth, about 8 to 10 minutes.

Place the dough in a greased bowl, turn to grease the top. Cover and let rise until doubled in size, about 1 hour.

Punch the dough down and turn out onto a lightly floured board. Divide into 4 equal parts, set 2 pieces aside. Roll 2 pieces of dough into ropes about 12 inches long; twist them together and tuck the ends under to seal. Place in a greased 8½x4½x2¾-inch loaf pan. Repeat with the remaining 2 pieces of dough to form a second loaf. Cover and let rise in a warm place until doubled in size, about 1 hour.

Preheat the oven to 400°. Bake for 30 minutes or until done.

TIPS & TRICKS:

- Hot water will kill the active yeast; don't let your water get too hot.
- You may be able to use the dough hook on your electric mixer for kneading. I made this in the pre-Kitchen Aid mixer days, so I kneaded by hand.

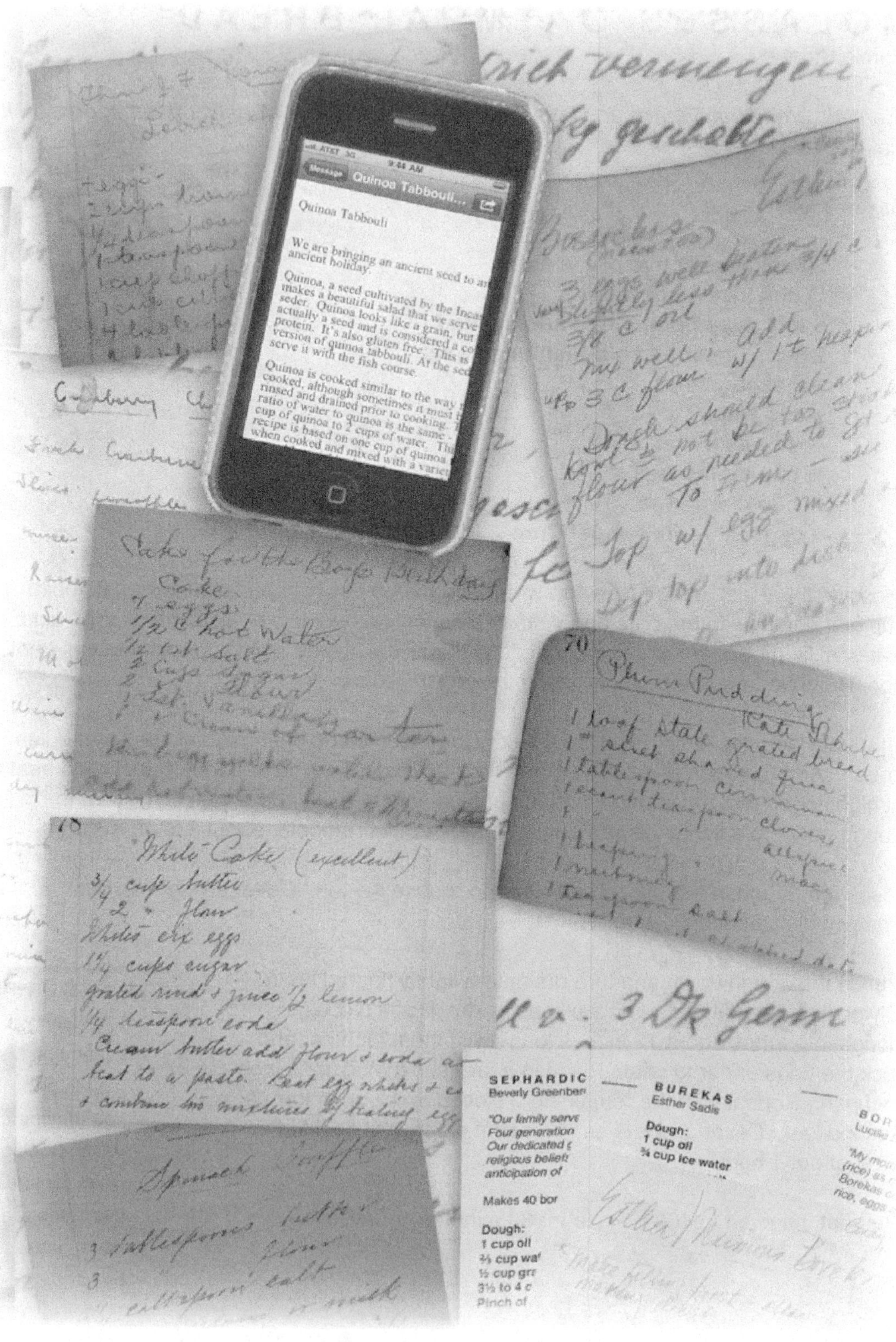
Quinoa Tabbouli...
Quinoa Tabbouli
We are bringing an ancient seed to an ancient holiday.
"White Cake (excellent)
SEPHARDIC
BUREKAS
Esther Sadis
Dough:
1 cup oil
¾ cup ice water
Makes 40 bor
Dough:
1 cup oil

Coffee Cake to Quesado

While soup, bread, and fish concoctions may have deep roots in Jewish tradition, brunch is a decidedly recent Western invention. "Brunch," a portmanteau of breakfast and lunch, is only traceable back to the turn-of-the-century Britain or New York. Although we can provide no enlightening story about the history of brunch throughout Jewish civilization, the following recipes express a fascinating meeting point between Jewish, American, and contemporary culture.

Most of the recipes included here are like culinary chameleons, whimsical enough to be served throughout the day but best suited to the brunch category. Put out quesado as an appetizer or a side, snack on Esther Lee's Banana Bread with a mid-afternoon cup of coffee, whip up Laurie Koehler's Chile Rellenos casserole for a light dinner.

Most Seattle Sephardic meals feature quesado, a variation of the frittata. Omelet-like dishes are more prevalent in Sephardic cuisine due to the influence of regional customs and the availability of eggs, and the quesado came over with the Turkish and Rhodesli immigrants to Seattle. This savory dish, usually made with spinach, never misses a Shabbat luncheon. According to Kathy Barokas, the versatile meal can be served for virtually every meal, from breakfast to dinner.

More familiar to American brunch cuisine are the coffee cakes, blintzes, and pastries that came over with Ashkenazi immigrants. Lisa Kranseler shares sweet memories of her Polish grandmother, who intuitively divined desserts and hid them under tables and chairs until it was time to eat them.

These brunch items took on their own significance in America. Michelle Tesler contributes a humorous story about her cooking days as a young bride and the sour cream coffee cake she got from a magazine in 1978, which years later was attributed to a family heirloom recipe. Now her grown son serves it at his own coffee house. Marilyn Kremen offers the Dutch Babies recipe that originated in the early 1900s in Seattle, which has not only been carried on but is also a remedy for any quibbles that come to the table. And Janet Rose reveals the recipe for Pumpkin Tea Bread that originated with a friend's pioneer grandmother and was kept secret until it appeared on the front page of the *Washington Post*.

TIDBIT:

- ❖ In America, typical brunch fare consists of eggs, pancakes, breakfast meats, and coffee on lazy Sunday mornings, while in Israel, hordes of people gather in restaurants late Friday morning to feast on eggs, bread, olives, cheese, and salads.
- ❖ So Anglo is the word and concept of brunch that the Académie Française encourage French nationals to refrain from using it, preferring instead its own version, *le grand petit dejeuner.*

Wikipedia

TIDBIT:

- In a map titled, "The Prevalence of Large and Small Omelets," Gil Marks maps out the types of eggs that Mizrachi and Sephardic Jews historically prepared. He points out that "countries influenced by the Italian frittata tend to make large, skillet-sized omelets. Arabic-influenced countries follow the Arabic style of cooking small, fried omelet patties. Persians enjoy both." Who knew?

  Gil Marks. *Olive Trees and Honey.*

- For being such a commodity in the modern world, eggs were a rarity and a luxury until the late Middle Ages. This was partly due to a lack of chickens and to the focus on breeding the fowl. Chicken became a more popular dish around the fifteenth century due to a meat shortage, and henceforth eggs began appearing in traditional dishes like challah, kugels and blintzes, as well as on their own. Eggs were always more prominent in Sephardic cooking.

  Gil Marks. *Olive Trees and Honey.*

COFFEE CAKE TO QUESADO

YEASTED COFFEE CAKE FOR THE NEW YEAR

Lynn Wartnik

"My mother, Annette Cohen, made these cakes every year for Rosh Hashanah and the High Holy Day dinners that followed. The scent of the yeast rising and the cake baking reminds me of the wonderful mother I was lucky enough to have. And, as I make these cakes for the holidays, I feel very close to her. Today, my granddaughters help me knead the dough and roll it out. Tomorrow, maybe they will be teaching their children."

Makes 4 coffee cakes

1 12-ounce can evaporated milk
½ cup butter
½ cup plus 1 tablespoon sugar
2 packets active dry yeast (not rapid-rising)
¼ cup very warm water (not hot)
3 eggs
½ teaspoon salt
5 to 6 cups all-purpose unbleached flour, sifted, plus more for kneading

Heat the evaporated milk with the butter until the butter is melted, but don't boil. After the mixture has cooled, about 15 minutes, add ½ cup of the sugar. Set aside.

Dissolve the yeast and the remaining sugar into the water. Allow the yeast mixture to sit for 10 minutes.

Beat the eggs in a large bowl with the salt. Add the cooled milk mixture. Stir with a wooden spoon, add the yeast mixture, and stir again.

Add the flour, one cup at a time, to the above mixture. Turn the mixture out onto a floured board and knead well. When the dough is smooth and no longer sticking to the board, place it into a lightly greased bowl. Cover the dough with a tea towel and let rise in a warm spot for 45 minutes. When the volume of the dough has doubled, punch it down and cut into 4 equal sections. Let the dough rest 5 minutes before rolling out.

Filling:
1 cup butter, melted and divided
1⅓ cup brown sugar
1 cup granulated sugar
6 teaspoons ground cinnamon
1⅓ cup raisins
1⅓ cup raspberry jam
⅓ cup cinnamon-sugar, for sprinkling

To assemble each coffee cake, roll one section of the dough at a time on a floured surface into a 16-inch circle.

Generously brush the dough with 1/3 to 1/2 cup of the melted butter all the way to the edges. Sprinkle the dough with the sugars, cinnamon, and raisins. Drop teaspoons of jam next to each other to form a log on the lower quarter of the dough.

Flip the bottom flap over the jam; then roll the circle into a log, as you would a jelly roll.

Place some parchment paper on a baking sheet and transfer the coffee cake to the covered baking sheet. Turn the ends slightly to form a crescent shape.

Repeat the entire process three more times with the remaining pieces of dough.

Preheat the oven to 350°.

Allow the cake to rise for another 20 minutes. Slit (do not cut through) the dough in 5 or 6 places, brush with melted butter, sprinkle with cinnamon-sugar and put the cake on the middle rack of the oven. Bake for 30 minutes, until nicely browned.

TIPS & TRICKS:

- The cake can be made in advance and frozen until ready to use. Carefully and completely wrap the cake before freezing.
- To make cinnamon-sugar, combine ½ cup of sugar with 1 tablespoon of cinnamon.
- The dough is perfect for cinnamon rolls. Brush the dough with butter and sprinkle the sugars, cinnamon, and raisins, if desired, over the dough and roll up like a jelly roll. Slice the roll into 1½-inch pieces and place each slice, cut-side down, into a well-buttered 9-inch cake pan, leaving just ½-inch between pieces. Let the rolls rise for 20 minutes, brush with melted butter, sprinkle with cinnamon sugar, then bake for 25 to 30 minutes until nicely browned.

SOUR CREAM COFFEE CAKE

Michele Tesler

"*When I got married in 1978, my mother bought me a subscription to* Bon Appetite *magazine, as well as an 8-week session of cooking classes with a contributing editor to the magazine. Each week I tried at least one new recipe from the magazine. This Sour Cream Coffee Cake recipe is from one of the issues published that year. It instantly became a favorite of our family and friends, and I made it frequently. Years later, my mother forgot the origin of the recipe and actually claimed once it was an 'old family recipe.' Living in Seattle since 1985, it has become a tradition at our break the fast meal. More recently, it can be found served daily at the Slow Train Café, a coffee house in Oberlin, Ohio, opened by our son Zach. But you don't have to travel that far for this delicious cake...you can make it in your own kitchen!*"

Makes one 10-inch coffee cake

3 cups flour
1½ teaspoons baking powder
1½ teaspoons baking soda
¼ teaspoon salt
1½ cups butter, room temperature
1½ cups sugar
3 eggs
1½ cups sour cream
2½ tablespoons vanilla, divided
¾ cup firmly packed brown sugar
¾ cup chopped walnuts (optional)
1½ teaspoons cinnamon
2 tablespoons water
Powdered sugar

Preheat the oven to 325°. Butter a 10-inch tube pan.

Sift together the flour, baking powder, baking soda, and salt and set aside.

In a large bowl, combine the butter and sugar and beat until fluffy. Add the eggs, one at a time, beating well after each addition. Blend in the sour cream and ½ tablespoon of the vanilla. Gradually add the dry ingredients to the wet ingredients and beat well.

For the nut topping, combine the brown sugar, walnuts, and cinnamon in a small bowl.

Spread a third of the thick batter into the prepared pan and sprinkle with half of the nut mixture. Repeat. Add the remaining third of batter.

Mix the remaining 2 tablespoons of vanilla with the water and spoon over the cake.

Bake for 60 to 70 minutes. Cool the cake for 10 minutes before removing from the pan. Dust the cake with powdered sugar.

ESTHER LEE'S BANANA BREAD

Esther Sadis

Makes one 9x5-inch loaf

2 ripe bananas
1½ cups sugar
2 eggs
½ cup vegetable oil
1¾ cups flour
1 teaspoon baking soda
1 teaspoon salt
¼ cup plus 1 tablespoon buttermilk
1 teaspoon vanilla
1 cup pecans or walnuts, chopped

Preheat the oven to 325°. Grease a 9x5-inch loaf pan.

In a large bowl, mash the bananas. Beat in the sugar, eggs, and oil.

Sift together the flour, baking soda, and salt. Mix with the banana mixture. Add the vanilla and buttermilk, then stir in the nuts.

Pour into the loaf pan and bake for 70 to 80 minutes, until the top is golden brown and split. Cool on wire rack for 20 minutes before removing from the pan.

PUMPKIN TEA BREAD

Janet and Fil Rose

"A nurse from Minnesota whom Janet worked with brought this wonderful bread to work. Everyone wanted the recipe. She said she could not give it out because it was a family secret. Her pioneer grandmother had passed it down in the family and asked that it be kept a secret family recipe.

"When Janet covered for her at the hospital during a long vacation, Janet's friend gave her the recipe, but made her promise that it not be given to anyone else. Janet kept her promise until the recipe appeared on the front page of the Washington Post *several years later when Joan Mondale had a tea in the Vice Presidential Mansion. The newspapers quoted Joan as saying it was an old Minnesota recipe. The part of the recipe that makes it really special is that it uses fresh pumpkin. It is a little more work, but well worth it.*

"So now it can be yours just as it has become a traditional holiday recipe for our family. Janet baked it with our children, and now our daughter bakes it with her two young children."

Makes 2 loaves

1½ cups sugar
1 teaspoon baking soda
¼ teaspoon baking powder
½ teaspoon cinnamon
1 teaspoon ground cloves
1 teaspoon nutmeg
¾ teaspoon salt
1⅔ cups unbleached flour, sifted
2 large eggs
½ cup vegetable oil
1 cup pumpkin, freshly baked (canned can also be used)
¼ cup water

Preheat the oven to 350°. Grease 2 loaf pans.

Sift together the sugar, baking soda, baking powder, cinnamon, cloves, nutmeg, salt, and flour. Add the eggs, oil, pumpkin, and water, and blend with a mixer. Pour the mixture into the 2 pans and bake for 50 to 60 minutes, until a toothpick inserted into the middle comes out clean. Cool in the pan on a wire rack.

TIPS & TRICKS:

❖ For freshly baked pumpkin, use a sugar pie pumpkin. Place the pumpkin in foil and bake at 375° for 1 hour or longer, if necessary. Cut the pumpkin in half and take out the seeds. Then scoop out the flesh and put it in a food processor for a few seconds to purée. Any leftovers can be frozen.

GRANDMA ROSE MOINESTER'S STRUDEL

Lisa Kranseler with help from mother, Cindy Coopersmith, and Aunt Deanna Albert

"My Grandma Rose was very special as all grandmothers are, but my memories of her were strictly related to her cooking, except for her pinches on the cheeks to us kids and calling us, 'mammashaina' or 'mishuggah.'

"Grandma Rose lived on a farm in Poland and was one of 7 siblings (2 boys, 5 girls). The family observed the Jewish religion, but was not particularly religious; luckily they left Poland, moving to Montreal, before the deep onset of Nazism.

"The kind of food my grandmother cooked was a heavy meal of mostly white-looking food, kosher chickens, stuffed cabbage, and potatoes. In those days, there was no knowledge or concern about fat content or cholesterol or any emphasis on nutrition. However, I sure can remember some of the old-time Jewish food, kugel, noodles, and especially the baked goods she loved to make. Grandma Rose was a natural, intuitive baker, who whipped her own meringue and would hide her delicious cakes under chairs or tables to save for dessert after dinner. My mother tells me she was very adept at finding them and dipping her finger to taste the sweetness of the creamy icing.

"Grandma Rose cooked alone in the old-fashioned kitchen of her home in Brooklyn and always brought her baking specialties to my family when she visited or babysat and even made them with us when we lived in New City, New York (Rockland County).

"My memories, and those of my brothers, Jeff and Steven, of Grandma Rose baking are quite vivid, particularly the fantastic aromas emanating from the kitchen, which would fill the whole house. I also can visualize her rolling out the dough with a makeshift roller or stick of wood, as she would never spend money on a rolling pin. She specialized in strudels, rugelach, mandelbreit, and noodle pudding. And each year, at Purim time, a box arrived in the mail filled with Grandma Rose's hamentashens. They were the best and didn't last long in our home.

"The absolute highlight of the year was when my parents took their annual vacation away from us kids, and my grandparents would come to stay with us. Of course we had to endure the very early dinners at 4:00 p.m., right when we came home from school, but it was so worth it, because we knew there would always be a special surprise that my Grandma had prepared.

"My favorite of all was her Everything Cake. This was when she called to us to bring out everything onto the kitchen counter that had anything to do with baking. It was so much fun, like a party. There was much giggling and fun as we took things out that we knew she wouldn't put in her cake, but we wanted to try to get her a bit excited. When all was said and done, she put in a 'little of this and a little of that' and voila, an hour later we had the most

delectable cake, a perfect delight, sometimes with coconut, M&M's, nuts, chocolate chips, bits of candy bars, raisins, or any combination, and sometimes maybe even all, of these.

"We cannot replicate her Everything Cake to the tee, but a little bit of Grandma Rose will always live on as my family has now instilled the tradition of making hamentashen each Purim and sending them to out-of-town family members. Two of our children enjoy cooking; they both have Grandma Rose's instinctive ability to create great food without an exact recipe. Our third child loves to eat the foods his brother and sister produce and we know he, too, will find time in the kitchen to experiment as well.

"Although I am relegated to sous-chef and known more as a cook than the chefs my kids claim name to, I do not mind. I know the traditions of my Grandma Rose will carry on, her recipes modernized with today's foodie in mind."

Makes 4 strudels

Dough:
2½ cups flour
½ teaspoon baking powder
¼ cup sugar
1 egg
½ cup oil
½ cup lukewarm water

Sift the flour, baking powder, and sugar into a mixing bowl. Add the egg, oil, and water and beat until the mixture forms a soft dough. Cover with a tea towel and let stand in a warm place for 1 hour.

Filling:
1 15-ounce package seedless raisins
½ orange, unpeeled
½ lemon, unpeeled
½ cup sugar
3 tablespoons seedless black raspberry jam
3 teaspoons cornflake crumbs or walnuts, chopped

Prepare the filling by mixing together the raisins, orange, lemon, sugar, and jam in a food processor and blending well so the citrus peels are chopped finely.

For Brushing and Sprinkling:
Canola oil
Cinnamon
Sugar
Powdered sugar

Preheat the oven to 400°.

Divide the dough into four pieces and roll each piece on a well-floured board until it is paper thin. Brush with oil and sprinkle lightly with your desired amount of cinnamon and sugar.

Spread one-fourth of the filling over the lower quarter of each sheet of dough. Sprinkle with one-fourth of the cornflake crumbs or chopped walnuts. Roll each sheet from the bottom up in a jelly roll fashion.

Arrange the strudels on a baking sheet and brush the top with oil and sprinkle with additional cinnamon and sugar. With a sharp knife, slash the top of each strudel at 1-inch intervals.

Bake for 15 minutes then reduce the oven temperature to 375°. Continue baking for 10 to 15 minutes longer, until golden brown. Remove the strudel from the oven, dust with powdered sugar, and cut into individual servings.

TIPS & TRICKS:

- The strudel was always delicious, but the recipe varied depending on what Grandma Rose had around the house. You can use nuts, raisins, or any kind of jam you prefer in the filling.

DANISH APPLE PASTRY BARS

Esther Lipson

Makes 3 dozen

2½ cups flour
1 teaspoon salt
1 cup shortening
1 egg, divided
⅔ cup milk (slightly less)
1 cup corn flakes
8 cups Granny Smith apples, peeled and sliced (about 4 large apples)
¾ cup (or less) sugar
1 teaspoon cinnamon
1 cup powdered sugar, sifted
4 to 5 teaspoons milk

Preheat the oven to 375°.

Combine the flour and salt in a medium-sized mixing bowl. Cut in the shortening. Beat the egg yolk in a measuring cup and add enough milk to make ⅔ cup liquid. Mix well and add to the flour mixture.

On a floured surface, roll half the dough into a 17x12-inch rectangle to fit into and up the sides of a 15½x10½x1-inch jelly roll pan. Sprinkle with the corn flakes and top with the apples, sugar, and cinnamon. Roll out the remaining dough and place over the apples. Seal the edges and cut a slit in the top. Beat the egg white until frothy and brush over the dough.

Bake for 50 minutes. Combine the powdered sugar with the milk and drizzle over the warm pastries. Cut into squares.

THE BREAKFAST – FOR – DINNER APPLE PANCAKE

David Masin

"One Sunday night, not too long ago, my parents invited us over for dinner. A typical Sunday night dinner would normally consist of chicken or chili or reservations at a favorite Chinese restaurant. This particular Sunday night, my mom decided to make this cinnamony-sweet apple pancake instead. Our son, 2 years old at the time, was quite confused by the idea of breakfast foods being served for dinner. He stared at the food on his plate and said, 'This is so silly.' Meanwhile, he took one bite and loved it. Since then, we've been calling it the 'breakfast-for-dinner apple pancake.'"

Serves 12 to 14

1 cup flour
1 cup milk
¼ teaspoon vanilla
4 eggs
½ cup dark brown sugar
½ cup sugar
¼ cup plus 1 tablespoon cinnamon
½ cup butter
4 Granny Smith apples (peeled, cored, and thinly sliced)

Preheat the oven to 400°.

In a mixing bowl, add the flour, milk, vanilla, and eggs. Mix well.

In another bowl, mix the brown sugar, sugar, and ¼ cup of the cinnamon

Put the butter and remaining tablespoon of the cinnamon in a 10x15-inch glass cooking casserole dish and place in the oven. When the butter is completely melted, remove the dish from the oven and add the apples to cover the bottom; coat the apples well with the cinnamon-butter mixture. Pour the batter over the apples, then sprinkle the entire surface with the cinnamon-sugar mixture.

Cook for approximately 40 minutes, until the edges are golden to dark brown. Let it cool for a few minutes before serving.

DUTCH BABIES

Marilyn Kremen

"Even though this recipe was created at Manca's restaurant in Seattle during the early part of the 1900s, many of us have carried on their tradition. I have made Dutch Babies for my family since our children were little. We used to have the little grade school kids come for breakfast and the tradition continued through high school and college. Everyone loves Dutch Babies in the morning with just a sprinkle of powdered sugar and a squeeze of lemon juice. It has been proven that families stay happier with this wonderful breakfast or brunch, as it is hard to be sad, mad, or bad when Dutch Babies are rising in the oven and everyone is anticipating the delicious taste – simply, a little bit of heaven. As our first grandchild, Oliver, starts to appreciate food when his teeth come in, Dutch Babies will definitely be one of his first really big bites!"

Makes 3 to 6 servings

The proportion of ingredients varies by the size of the cast iron pan used to make the Dutch Babies. The following chart will help you determine the quantities needed to make the perfect Dutch Baby. Pour water by the quart into a pan to determine the capacity of the pan.

PAN SIZE	BUTTER	EGGS	MILK AND FLOUR
2 to 3 quart	**¼ cup**	**3**	**¾ cup each**
3 to 4 quart	**⅓ cup**	**4**	**1 cup each**
4 to 4½ quart	**½ cup**	**5**	**1¼ cups each**
4½ to 5 quart	**½ cup**	**6**	**1½ cups each**

Lemon wedges
Powdered sugar

Preheat the oven to 425°. Place the butter in the pan and melt in the oven.

In a blender or food processor, mix the eggs on high speed for 1 minute. With the motor running, gradually pour in the milk, then slowly add the flour, continuing to blend for 30 seconds.

Remove the pan from the oven and pour in the batter. Return the pan to the oven and bake until the pancake is puffy and well-browned, about 20 to 25 minutes, depending on the pan size. Do not open the oven during cooking or the pancake will not rise properly.

Remove from the oven and dust with powdered sugar and squeeze lemon juice over the Dutch Baby. Cut into wedges and serve.

SARAH BLOOM GOODMAN'S COTTAGE CHEESE PANCAKES

Darcy Goodman

"These pancakes can be whipped up in no time and are fantastic."

Makes ten 3-inch pancakes

3 eggs, well beaten
1 cup of cottage cheese, put through a sieve
¼ cup flour
¼ teaspoon salt
3 tablespoons butter, softened
Maple syrup or jam, for serving

Mix together the eggs, cottage cheese, flour, and salt. Add 2 tablespoons of the butter and mix again.

Heat a nonstick skillet and melt the remaining butter. Pour the desired amount of batter into the skillet and cook until bubbles start to form on the surface. Flip the pancakes and continue cooking until golden brown. Serve with maple syrup or your choice of jam.

GRANDMA RUTHIE'S FAMOUS BLINTZ PANCAKES

Carin Sulman Jacobson

"There was never a sleepover at Grandma Ruthie's when her famous blintzes weren't the first of the morning treat. Each of her beloved grandchildren loves the blintzes she still makes, and today they are serving them to their own children."

2 servings

½ cup flour
¼ teaspoon salt
2 eggs
1 cup milk
Butter
Raspberry jam
Powdered sugar

Combine the flour and salt in a mixing bowl. Beat the eggs lightly, add the milk, and mix. Gradually add the egg mixture to the flour, beating until smooth.

Heat butter in a small to medium-sized frying pan over medium heat until sizzling. Pour about ⅓ cup of the batter and spread by tilting the pan back and forth. When the pancake starts to bubble, flip it over gently. One side should be slightly brown. Continue cooking until other side is browned and remove from heat.

Spread one side with raspberry jam (or another variety) and roll the crepe into a log and sprinkle with powdered sugar. Serve hot.

CHEESE BLINTZES

Tina Lippman Kahn

Makes 24 blintzes

Filling:
1 cup cottage cheese
8 ounces cream cheese
1 egg, well beaten
2 tablespoons butter, melted
2 tablespoons sugar
¼ cup golden raisins (optional)
1 teaspoon vanilla

Blend the cottage cheese, cream cheese, egg, butter, sugar, raisins, if desired, and vanilla together. Set aside or refrigerate if not using immediately.

Blintzes:
1½ cups flour
¼ teaspoon salt
4 eggs, beaten
2 tablespoons butter, melted, plus more for frying and brushing
2 cups milk
Sour cream
Fruit preserves

Combine the flour and salt in a mixing bowl. Add the eggs and mix well. Add the butter, then gradually add the milk to make a smooth batter.

Heat an 8-inch frying pan over medium heat and melt 1 teaspoon butter. Add 2 tablespoons of the batter, tilting the pan to spread the batter. Cook the pancake until slightly golden brown on the bottom then remove to a paper towel. Repeat with the remaining batter.

Place 1 tablespoon of the filling in the center of the browned side and fold the blintz from opposite sides into an envelope shape. Cool and refrigerate. Repeat this process with the rest of the batter and the filling.

When ready to serve, brush each completed blintz with some additional melted butter and place in a buttered skillet. Fry until golden brown on all sides.

Serve with your choice of sour cream and fruit preserves.

TIPS & TRICKS:

❖ If you aren't serving the blintzes immediately, place them in a 9x13-inch glass baking dish to be reheated later in a 350° oven for 20 minutes.

GESCHMERTE MATZO

Rhoda S. Lewis

Makes 6 matzo sheets

2 pints cottage cheese
1 cup sugar, plus additional for topping
1 teaspoon vanilla
1 teaspoon salt
½ cup raisins
4 eggs
6 sheets matzo
Butter
Cinnamon

Preheat the oven to 350°.

Mix the cottage cheese, sugar, vanilla, salt, raisins, and eggs together.

Rinse each sheet of the matzo lightly with water and lay them on a jelly roll pan.

Spread the mixed ingredients over the matzo. Dot each piece of matzo with butter and sprinkle with cinnamon and sugar.

Bake for 20 minutes. Cut into squares before serving.

TIPS & TRICKS:

- For a crunchy topping, you can put pieces of rinsed matzo on top of the cottage cheese mixture, dot with butter, sprinkle with cinnamon and sugar, and bake.
- You can also bake this in a 7x11-inch glass baking dish.

FRENCH TOAST BREAD PUDDING

Jo Jassny

Serves 10 to 12

8 1½-inch thick slices challah, crusts removed
4 eggs
1 cup milk
1 teaspoon sugar
1 pinch salt
2 tablespoons orange juice
½ teaspoon vanilla
1 tablespoon butter, melted
Powdered sugar
Syrup

Place the bread in a well buttered 9x13-inch pan. Blend the eggs, milk, sugar, salt, orange juice, vanilla, and butter. Pour the mixture over the bread. Cover and refrigerate overnight.

When ready to bake, preheat the oven to 350°. Bake for 1 hour. Sprinkle with powdered sugar, drizzle with syrup, and serve.

SPINACH QUESADO

Jeanie Alhadeff

Serves 16 to 20

1 40-ounce bag spinach, stems removed and coarsely chopped
2½ cups feta cheese, crumbled
3 cups Parmesan cheese, grated
2 cups small curd cottage cheese
3 sheets matzo, briefly soaked in water to soften, then squeezed dry
14 eggs, beaten
2 tablespoons olive oil
2 tablespoons butter, for dotting
½ to 1 cup Parmesan cheese, shredded, for sprinkling

Preheat the oven to 350°.

Mix the spinach, feta, 3 cups of the Parmesan cheese, and cottage cheese together.

Mix the matzo and beaten eggs together, pour over the spinach mixture and blend.

Put the olive oil in a 10x15-inch pan or glass dish and tip the pan until the bottom is covered with the oil. Pour the spinach and egg mixture into the pan. Dot with the butter and sprinkle with the desired amount of cheese.

Bake for 45 to 60 minutes, until the top is golden brown. Cut into squares and serve warm.

TOMATO QUESADO

Jeanie Alhadeff

Serves 16 to 20

2 28-ounce cans whole tomatoes, drained
1 tablespoon plus 1 teaspoon oil
1 teaspoon salt
10 eggs
2 sheets matzo, soaked and squeezed dry
1 pint cottage cheese
⅓ cup each grated Parmesan, Romano, and feta cheese

Preheat the oven to 375°.

Place the tomatoes, 1 teaspoon of the oil, and salt in a large pan over medium heat and bring to a simmer. Crush the tomatoes coarsely continue to simmer and cook until the tomatoes soften and the mixture is smooth. This could take about 1 hour.

In a bowl, beat the eggs. Add the matzo, cottage cheese, Parmesan, Romano, and feta cheeses and mix well with your hands. (This must be done with your hands or it won't taste right). You may want to add some additional cheese.

Pour 1 tablespoon of the oil into a 10x15-inch baking dish and heat in the oven until it is hot. Pour in both the tomato and egg mixtures and bake for 1 hour and 10 minutes, until brown around edges.

ZUCCHINI QUESADO

Kathy Barokas

"My mother always offered to make this delicious family favorite whenever we traveled to the ocean or somewhere else. It can be reheated and served anytime for breakfast, brunch, lunch, snack, or a light dinner."

Serves 10 to 16

3 small zucchinis, unpeeled and grated
1 carrot, peeled and grated
½ teaspoon salt
1¼ cup Parmesan cheese
1 cup crumbled feta cheese
1 cup matzo meal (or 3 slices white bread, torn into pieces)
5 to 6 eggs, well beaten
⅓ cup oil
Flour, for dusting

Preheat the oven to 350°.

Squeeze the zucchini until all of the liquid is released and place it into a large bowl. Add the grated carrot. Mix in 1 cup of the Parmesan cheese and the feta cheese. Add the matzo meal (or the bread) and the eggs and mix well.

Pour the oil into a 9x13-inch glass dish and heat the dish in the oven. Sprinkle just a bit of flour into the dish, then pour in the zucchini mixture. Sprinkle the top with the remaining ¼ cup of Parmesan cheese.

Bake for 35 to 40 minutes, until the top of the egg mixture springs back.

SERBIAN EGGS

Doreen Alhadeff

"This has been my go-to recipe for years for brunch. It is always a hit."

Serves 12

7 eggs
1 pound jack cheese, grated
1 cup Bisquick
½ cup butter, melted and cooled a bit
16 ounces small curd cottage cheese
1 cup whole milk
1 or 2 4-ounce cans mild diced green chilies, drained (optional)

Preheat the oven to 350°. Grease a 9x13-inch baking dish.

Combine the eggs, jack cheese, Bisquick, butter, cottage cheese, milk, and chilies, and pour into the baking dish.

Bake 40 to 50 minutes, until casserole no longer jiggles in the middle.

SCRUMPTIOUS EGGS

Lynne Shutt

"I inherited this recipe from a friend when we hosted a brunch and bridal shower together. We served it with fruit and fresh pastries, and it was the perfect brunch menu. Now this is my 'go-to' egg recipe. It's fantastic that I can do most of the prep work the day before and add the eggs at the last minute, then bake. It is such a simple recipe with such delicious flavors."

Serves 10

1½ pounds Monterey jack cheese, shredded and divided
½ cup butter, melted
1⅛ pounds fresh mushrooms, sliced
1 large onion, finely chopped
11 eggs, beaten
2⅔ cups milk
¾ cup flour
1½ tablespoons parsley, chopped
Salt and white pepper, to taste

Place half of the cheese in the bottom of a buttered 9x13-inch glass dish.

Melt the butter in a large fry pan and sauté the mushrooms and onion until tender. Transfer the vegetables so they cover the cheese in the baking dish. Put the remaining cheese over top of the vegetables, cover, and refrigerate until ready to bake.

Preheat the oven to 350°.

When ready to bake, beat the eggs with the milk, flour, and parsley. Season to taste then pour evenly over the casserole. Bake for 45 minutes. Cover with foil and let it sit for 15 minutes before serving.

CHILI RELLENOS CASSEROLE

Laurie Koehler

Serves 8

1 cup half-and-half (or any kind of milk)
2 eggs
⅓ cup flour
3 4-ounce cans mild whole green chilies, split, seeded, and drained on paper towels
¾ cup Monterey jack cheese, shredded
¾ cup medium cheddar cheese, shredded
1 8-ounce can tomato sauce or salsa

Preheat the oven to 350°. Butter a 9x9-inch glass dish.

Beat the half-and-half, eggs, and flour until smooth.

Mix the Monterey jack and cheddar cheeses together. Reserve ½ cup for sprinkling on the top.

Layer one-third of the chilies, ½ cup of the cheese mixture, one-third of the egg mixture, repeating the process two more times. Top the third layer with the tomato sauce and sprinkle with the reserved cheese mixture.

Bake for 1¼ hours.

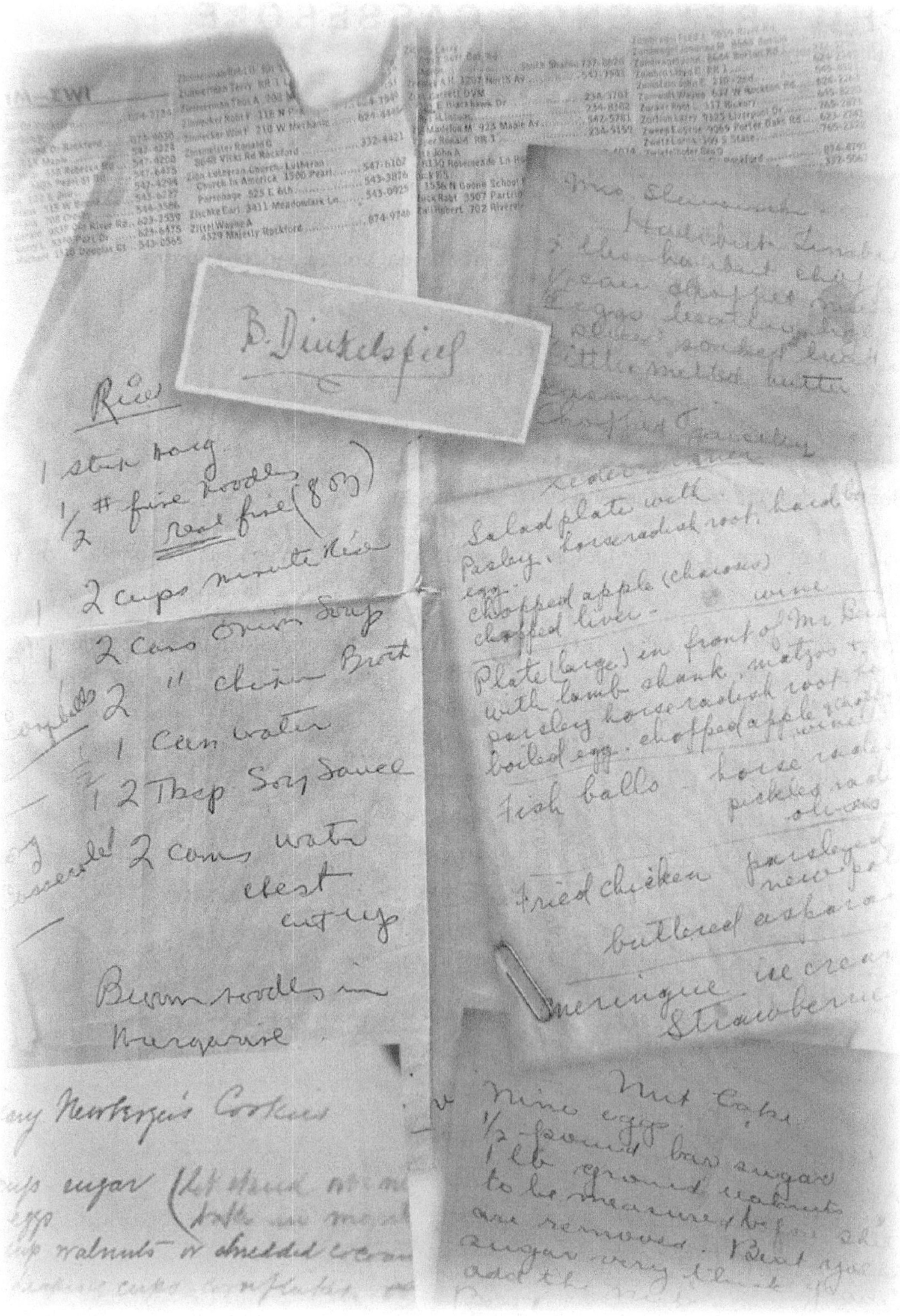
B. Dinkelspiel
Rice
2 cups minute Rice
2 Cans Onion Soup
1 Can water
2 Tbsp Soy Sauce
Salad plate with
chopped apple (charoses)
chopped liver
Plate (large) in front of Mr
with lamb shank, matzos
boiled egg
Fish balls
Fried chicken
buttered asparagus
meringue
Strawberries
Nut Cake
Nine eggs
1 lb ground walnuts

Cole Slaw to Niçoise

The creators of this cookbook often returned to the same questions during its production: What is Jewish food? What is Pacific Northwest food? What is a maven? What is a foodie?

As much as we took out our proverbial knives, razor-sharp and slightly damp, to cut these categories cleanly, it became a futile exercise. However, the distinction between maven and foodie in the context of time and place comes through clearest in this chapter.

All one need do is open up a classic cookbook, like Mrs. Simon Kander's *The Settlement Cookbook*, to see what has happened to salad over the decades. Salad recipes from what we might consider the maven generation rely on a pantry full of ingredients spurned or snubbed by today's foodies, like mayonnaise (as in, Boiled Mayonnaise Dressing) vinegar (white, that is), and gelatin (as in, Chicken Salad Mold or – wait for it – Liver Aspic). Canned food was instrumental: canned pears, mixed with cream cheese, grapes, French dressing, and mayonnaise made the crowd-pleaser, Bunch of Grapes Salad. Top some bananas with Boiled Mayonnaise Dressing and whipped cream, and voila, there you have Banana Salad.

Perhaps a day will come when our descendants will laugh and clutch their hearts when they think about our salads. But we think they're fabulous. We have our throwbacks to the old days, like Judy Schocken's Beet and Herring Salad and Beverly Wolfers' Cole Slaw, handed down from her mother-in-law Hilde, who came to America from Germany via Guatemala City and the good graces of a Montana dude ranch. Cynthia Flash Hemphill takes the painstaking work of making dolmas (stuffed grape leaves) and revises the traditional Sephardic dish into a tantalizing – and easy – salad.

Today's foodies go on adventures with international flavors and compelling combinations. Not to mention that the food industry, for all its flaws, has provided us with rare and imported fruits, a spectrum of exotic vinegars, oils, grains, cheeses, herbs, and spices, making today's kitchen something of a playground.

A perfect example is Brooke Benaroya Dickson's Persimmon and Pomegranate Salad, a "simple" recipe that utilizes exotic fruit, a variety of greens, and sherry vinegar. (But simpler than Banana Salad? The jury's still out.) Mary Anne Stusser Martin, the "salad queen," combines greens, strawberries, figs, goat cheese, and green beans with a zesty balsamic dressing, while Marleen Alhadeff doctors up basic lettuce with an emulsion of tarragon oil, bleu cheese, anchovy paste, and garlic. The abundance of available resources, just a salad fork's distance away, combined with a sense of adventure for flavors and ingredients, put today's foodies on the salad frontier.

The foodie salad recipes here are also the most divergent from our historical theme, but their presence on our table, meal after meal, holiday after holiday, makes them newly traditional and just as revered as the old timers.

COLE SLAW TO NIÇOISE

BEET AND HERRING SALAD

Judy Schocken

Serves 8 to 10

2 cups cooked beets
1 12-ounce jar of herring in wine sauce
½ cup walnuts
1 granny smith or sweeter apple, peeled and cored
1 to 2 Yukon Gold or red potatoes, cooked until fork-tender
2 eggs, hard boiled
2 dill pickles
½ sweet onion
¼ cup parsley
½ to ¾ cup mayonnaise, depending on your taste

Dice the beets, herring, walnuts, apple, potatoes, eggs, pickles, onions, and parsley. Combine with the mayonnaise to blend. It can be thinned out with pickle juice and yogurt, if desired.

GREEN BEANS, WALNUT, AND FETA SALAD

Bel Borromeo

Serves 6 to 8

1½ pounds haricot vert (French green beans), ends trimmed
¾ cup olive oil
½ cup fresh mint leaves, packed
¼ cup white wine vinegar
¾ teaspoon salt
½ teaspoon garlic, minced
¼ teaspoon pepper, freshly ground
1 cup walnuts, toasted and coarsely chopped
1 cup red onion, finely chopped
1 cup feta cheese, crumbled

Bring 4 quarts of salted water to a boil in a 6-quart saucepan over medium heat. Add the green beans and cook until crisp and still green, about 4 minutes. Drain, then plunge into ice water to stop the cooking process. Drain and pat dry.

Combine the oil, mint, vinegar, salt, garlic, and pepper in a processor and blend.

Arrange the cooked beans on a platter. Sprinkle with the nuts, red onion, and feta cheese. Drizzle the dressing over the top and serve.

ROASTED BEETS WITH MACADAMIA NUT PESTO

Leslie Huppin

Makes 6 servings

1 pound beets, skins on, stems removed, and scrubbed
½ cup plus 1 tablespoon extra-virgin olive oil
1 cup fresh basil leaves, loosely packed
2 cloves garlic
1 tablespoon ginger root, peeled and roughly chopped
¼ cup macadamia nuts
2 tablespoons sea salt, divided
Freshly ground pepper, to taste
1 cup feta cheese, crumbled
½ cup raisins

Preheat the oven to 400°.

Coat the beets with 1 tablespoon of the olive oil and season with 1 tablespoon of the salt. Place the beets on a sheet of aluminum foil and fold the foil around them. Roast for approximately 1½ hours, until beets are almost tender when pierced with a toothpick.

Remove the beets from the oven and let them steam in the foil for an additional 30 minutes. Remove the skins and slice the beets into desired shapes.

For the pesto, put the remaining ½ cup of olive oil, basil, garlic, ginger, macadamia nuts, and teaspoon of salt in the blender. Purée for about 10 seconds, until the ingredients are roughly smooth.

Heat a sauté pan over medium heat, add the beets and pesto, and cook until heated through, approximately 1 minute. Season with the pepper and arrange on individual plates or in a serving bowl. Sprinkle with the feta cheese and raisins.

HILDE'S 24-HOUR COLE SLAW

Beverly Wolfers

"Hilde Nathan Wolfers was born into a privileged banking family in Essen, Germany, in 1900. She married and had two sons. In 1939, they fled Germany and moved to Guatemala City where they had a much different life. She and her family lived in a shack and were too proud to ask any of her relatives for money. Coincidentally, an American family was visiting Guatemala, and they were looking for two young, Jewish men to help them at their dude ranch in West Yellowstone, Montana. That is how my husband and his brother entered the United States. Hilde finally followed, and when she was 60 years old, she got her first job in a hospital as a nurse's aide, where she won many awards for her service. She loved to cook foods from all countries, although her specialty was German cooking. This cole slaw is a recipe she used to make for our family celebrations."

Serves 10 to 12

1 3-pound head green cabbage
2 large carrots, shredded
3 green onions, chopped
½ cup green pepper, chopped
½ cup vinegar
½ cup salad oil
½ cup sugar
½ teaspoon salt
1 teaspoon dry mustard
1 teaspoon celery seed

Combine the cabbage, carrots, onions, and green peppers in a large bowl.

In a sauce pan, bring the vinegar, oil, sugar, salt, mustard, and celery seed to a boil for 3 minutes. Pour the dressing over the cabbage mixture and mix well. Refrigerate, covered, for at least 24 hours. The salad will keep for several days in the refrigerator. Before serving, be sure to drain off any extra dressing.

PERSIMMON AND POMEGRANANTE SALAD

Brooke Benaroya Dickson

"This fall salad is adapted from a recipe in Alice Water's, The Art of Simple Food. *It is a fall favorite in our house."*

Serves 8 to 10

1 shallot
2 tablespoons sherry vinegar
6 cups assorted fall greens (escarole, radicchio, endive, etc.)
6 ripe Fuyu persimmons
1 small pomegranate
Salt and pepper
5 tablespoons olive oil
½ cup walnuts, toasted

Mince the shallot and add to sherry vinegar with a little salt to macerate.

Tear the fall greens and place in a large salad bowl.

Slice the persimmons or cut them into narrow wedges. Remove the seeds from the pomegranate.

Whisk the olive oil with the vinegar and season with salt and pepper. Dress the leaves with some of the olive oil mixture and toss. Add the fruit and a bit more dressing and lightly toss again. Top with the toasted walnuts if desired.

TIPS & TRICKS:

❖ Round Fuyu persimmons are sweet and ready-to-eat when just barely softening. Their flesh is still firm, making them great for salads (the other common variety, hachiya, have a pointy tip and are astringent until extremely soft and custard-like').

NOT YOUR SIMPLE GREEN SALAD

Mary Anne Stusser Martin

"I am known as the 'salad queen' among my family and friends. Whenever we have potlucks, I bring the salad, and it is never a 'simple green!' Here is my favorite combination."

Serves 6 to 8

Salad:
6 cups mixed baby greens
2 cups arugula
1 cup strawberries, sliced
1 cup fresh figs, diced (may substitute dates)
1 cup fresh green beans, diced
4 ounces goat cheese, crumbled
½ cup slivered almonds
Maple syrup

Place the baby greens, arugula, strawberries, figs, green beans, and goat cheese in a large bowl.

Pour a thin layer of maple syrup into a sauté pan and add the almonds. Sauté over medium heat, stirring constantly, until the syrup is absorbed into the almonds. Remove from heat and spread the almonds evenly in a single layer on baking sheet. Freeze for 15 minutes. Crumble the almonds and add them to the salad.

Balsamic Vinaigrette:
1 cup olive oil
½ cup balsamic vinegar
1 tablespoon Dijon mustard
1 tablespoon honey

Whisk together the olive oil, balsamic vinegar, Dijon mustard, and honey. Toss the salad with just enough dressing to coat.

TIPS & TRICKS:

- You can use almost any other fresh vegetable in this salad that you want

GRANDPA'S FAVORITE SALAD

Beverly Schoenfeld

"A light and refreshing salad!"

Serves 8

1/3 cup lemon juice
3/4 cup olive oil (less if you prefer)
1 teaspoon salt
Ground pepper
3 large cloves garlic, pressed
1 pint cherry tomatoes
1/3 cup slivered almonds, toasted
1/3 cup Jarlsberg cheese, grated
8 cups romaine lettuce, chopped

Mix the lemon juice, olive oil, salt, pepper, and garlic together and set aside for several hours.

Combine the cherry tomatoes, almonds, Jarlsberg cheese, and romaine in a large bowl. Just before serving, toss the salad with the dressing.

TARRAGON, BLEU CHEESE, AND ANCHOVY SALAD

Marleen Alhadeff

"This recipe was given to me by my mother-in-law, Joan Alhadeff. Our family savors the flavor of anchovies, and we just love this salad."

Serves 6

2/3 cup olive oil
1/3 cup tarragon vinegar
2 to 4 cloves garlic, minced (add more or less to your own taste)
1/2 tube anchovy paste
1 1/2 heads lettuce, cut into chunks
2 tablespoons bleu cheese, crumbled (add more if desired)
Freshly ground black pepper, to taste

In a blender mix the olive oil, tarragon vinegar, garlic, and anchovy paste.

Put the lettuce into a large salad bowl. Sprinkle with the bleu cheese.

Toss the salad with the desired amount of dressing. Season to taste with pepper.

TIPS & TRICKS:

- ❖ Consider using red leaf or romaine lettuce.

UNDER – THE – STARS SUKKOT SALAD

Miriam Coates

Serves 4

"At what point does a personal recipe transform into a family recipe? How many years must a dish be served for a holiday before it becomes a traditional dish? For my children, ages 7 and 9, Sukkot salad has been served under the stars in our sukkah for as long as they can remember.

"There is nothing significantly symbolic or historic about the salad other than it contains pomegranate seeds (for the 613 mitzvot and to honor the return of Persephone and Demeter's joy) and the bitter herb, parsley. However, it is a very attractive salad, easy to make, and perfect for young chefs."

4 cups mixed lettuces, including baby leaf variety
1 cucumber, peeled, halved lengthwise, and seeded
2 Satsumas or tangerines, peeled, separated into sections, and membrane removed
½ cup pomegranate seeds
1 or 2 radishes, sliced into ¼-inch pieces
½ cup parsley, finely chopped
1 lemon, juiced
¼ teaspoon extra virgin olive oil
Pinch of sea salt
Pepper, to taste
3 sprigs of chives, chopped, as a garnish

Wash and dry the lettuces, leaving baby leaves whole and tearing the others into a large bowl.

Cut the cucumber into ¼-inch slices and add to the lettuce mix. Add the orange sections and pomegranate seeds. Add the radishes and parsley.

Mix the lemon juice, olive oil, salt, and pepper to taste, then pour over the lettuce, vegetables, and fruits. Toss and garnish with the chives.

PANZANELLA SALAD

Julie Faison

"Panzanella is traditionally an Italian bread salad containing tomatoes, cucumbers, olives, or many other possible ingredients. Usually, it is served with grilled bread, but this salad is made with crunchy, garlic and herb-infused croutons. It is wonderful anytime of the year, but especially late summer when sweet, vine-ripened tomatoes are plentiful."

Serves 12 to 18

Croutons:
½ cup olive oil
2 large cloves garlic, minced
1 tablespoon herb mixture (see TIPS AND TRICKS)
8 cups peasant bread, crusts removed and cut into 1-inch cubes

Preheat the oven to 425°.

Mix the olive oil, garlic, and herbs in a small bowl.

Place the bread in a large bowl. Working quickly, pour the olive oil mixture over the bread, evenly incorporating as much of the mixture as possible. Transfer the croutons to a large baking sheet with sides.

Bake for 5 minutes, stir, and bake for another 5 minutes. Repeat until the croutons are nicely browned, about 15 to 20 minutes in total, being careful not to burn.

Dressing:
⅔ cup extra virgin olive oil
3 tablespoons red wine vinegar
⅓ cup fresh basil, finely chopped
1 large clove garlic, minced
¼ teaspoon salt
Pinch of freshly ground pepper

Combine the olive oil, vinegar, basil, garlic, salt, and pepper.

Salad:
6 cups cherry tomatoes, halved
1½ English cucumbers, unpeeled and cut into ¾-inch dice
1 large green pepper, cut into ¾-inch dice
¾ cup pitted kalamata olives, halved lengthwise
¼ cup capers, rinsed and drained, chopped
4 cups croutons
1 cup fresh basil leaves, rolled together lengthwise, then sliced into ¼-inch slices

In a large bowl, combine the tomatoes, cucumbers, green peppers, olives, and capers. Pour the dressing over the salad. Add the croutons and the basil, toss again.

TIPS & TRICKS:

- When stirring the croutons, shift them from the edge of the pan into the middle (and vise versa) to help bake more evenly.
- You can also add fresh mozzarella or feta cheese to this salad.
- The herb mixture can be made in larger quantities and used for other purposes. Try as a seasoning for chicken or combining with softened butter and garlic for garlic bread, or sprinkling over any number of green or pasta salads.
- Herb Mix Recipe:
  - 3 teaspoons Herbs de Provence
  - 1 teaspoon thyme
  - 1 teaspoon oregano
  - 1 teaspoon basil
  - 1 teaspoon rosemary
  - 1 teaspoon freshly ground pepper

QUINOA TABOULI

Carlyn Koch Steiner

"We are bringing an ancient seed to an ancient holiday. Quinoa, a seed cultivated by the Incas, makes a beautiful salad that we serve at the Seder. Quinoa looks like a grain, but it is actually a seed and is considered a complete protein. It's also gluten free. This is my version of quinoa tabouli. At the Seder we serve it with the fish course."

Makes 4 cups

1 cup quinoa
½ cup fresh lemon juice, divided
½ cup cucumber, peeled, salted, chopped, and patted dry
1 clove garlic, finely minced
½ cup tomato, seeded and chopped
½ cup green onion, chopped
½ cup parsley, chopped
2 tablespoons mint, chopped
2 teaspoons ground cumin
¼ cup good olive oil
Salt and pepper, to taste

Cook the quinoa according to packing instructions. When cooked, fluff and turn into a bowl. Add 3 tablespoons of the lemon juice to begin flavoring. Mix and cool the quinoa.

Mix the quinoa with the cucumber, garlic, tomato, green onion, parsley, mint, cumin, the remaining 5 tablespoons of the lemon juice, olive oil, salt, and pepper. Refrigerate for several hours, then taste, and re-season with salt, pepper, and a bit more lemon juice.

TIPS & TRICKS:

- Quinoa is cooked as rice is cooked, rinsed and drained before cooking. The ratio of water to quinoa is the same as rice, 1 cup of quinoa to 2 cups of water.
- The tabouli lends itself well to additions. Consider cilantro, avocado, toasted nuts, dried fruit, black beans, and, for heat, red pepper flakes.

DOLMAS SALAD

Cynthia Flash Hemphill

"This is an easy way to make dolmas without having to roll them up. It is good warm, although I prefer it room temperature or cold."

Serves 6 to 8

¼ cup pine nuts
½ cup green onions (white and pale green parts only), thinly sliced and divided
1 tablespoon olive oil
1½ cups long-grain white rice
2½ cups chicken broth (or vegetable broth, if preferred)
½ cup preserved grape leaves, chopped
¼ cup brine from grape leaves
¼ cup lemon juice
¼ cup raisins
¼ teaspoon pepper
¼ cup parsley, chopped
½ cup fresh dill, chopped
Lemon quarters, as a garnish (optional)

In a 4 to 6-quart pan over medium heat, stir the pine nuts and ¼ cup of the green onions in the oil until the nuts begin to brown and the onions are limp, about 5 minutes. Stir in the rice, chicken broth, grape leaves, ¼ cup of the brine, lemon juice, raisins, and pepper. Bring to a boil, then reduce heat to low, cover and simmer until liquid is absorbed and the rice is tender to the bite, 30 to 35 minutes.

Fluff the rice with a fork, stir in the parsley, dill, and remaining ¼ cup of the green onions. Mound the salad on a platter and garnish with lemon quarters, if desired.

PARTY – IN – YOUR – MOUTH SALAD

Iantha Sidell

"We serve this salad for Rosh Hashanah, but really, anytime you are having a crowd for an event, it is a perfect accompaniment to any meal."

Serves 16

4 cups wild rice
12 cups chicken broth
2 cups dried apricots, chopped
½ cup currants
½ cup dried cranberries
2 cups slivered almonds, toasted
1⅓ cups red onions, chopped
1 cup parsley, chopped
4 cloves garlic, minced
Salt and pepper, to taste

Cook the rice in the chicken broth according to the package directions, for at least 45 minutes, until the rice kernels pop open. Drain the rice and transfer to a large bowl. Mix the apricots, cranberries, and currants into the rice mixture then cool completely.

Mix the almonds, red onion, parsley, and garlic into the cooled rice.

Dressing:
¾ cup tarragon vinegar
Scant 3 tablespoons Dijon mustard
2 cups olive oil (or less if desired)

For the dressing, combine the vinegar and mustard in a bowl. Gradually whisk in the olive oil. Toss the rice with the preferred amount of dressing just before serving. Season to taste with salt and pepper.

TIPS & TRICKS:

- This recipe can easily be doubled for a big crowd.

ASIAN NOODLE SALAD

Andrea Lott

Serves 10 to 12

1 pound thin spaghetti or Rose Brand Chinese egg noodles
¼ cup double black soy sauce
¼ cup sesame oil
2 tablespoons sugar
1 tablespoon hot chili oil
2 tablespoons balsamic vinegar
½ cup sesame seeds, toasted
1 bunch green onions, thinly sliced as a garnish

Cook the spaghetti until al denté. Drain, rinse with cold water, and drain again to get as much water off the noodles as possible.

In a small bowl, mix the soy sauce, sesame oil, sugar, chili oil, and balsamic vinegar, dissolving the sugar. Pour the mixture over the noodles and mix well.

Add the sesame seeds and toss the noodles again. Garnish with the green onions.

TIPS & TRICKS:

- ❖ Make this into a one dish entrée by topping with grilled chicken and garnishing with red and yellow peppers and snap peas.
- ❖ Double black soy has a more intense flavor than traditional soy sauce and can be found at Uwajimaya in Seattle or any other Asian supermarket.

TUNA NIÇOISE PASTA SALAD

Mike Cheifetz

Serves 8 to 10

2 7-ounce cans tuna, packed in oil
2 cloves garlic, minced
1 red bell pepper, chopped
1 cup green olives with pimento or kalamata olives, if preferred
2 tablespoons capers, drained
1 lemon, juiced
1 15-ounce package of pasta, cooked (small shells, penne, farfalle, or other pasta of your choice)

Drain the tuna, reserving the oil from one can.

In a wok or sauté pan, sauté the garlic and peppers in the reserved tuna oil. Add the tuna, olives, and capers and heat through.

Add the cooked pasta to the tuna mixture. Pour the lemon juice over the entire mixture and toss to blend. This salad can be served warm or at room temperature.

Jewish Penicillin to the Borscht Belt

Eastern European Jewish immigrants saw America as the land of opportunity, but little did they imagine that their soups would be among their most noteworthy contributions. Few stories of impoverished beginnings result in such superstar status. Who could have predicted that some lowly beets would have an entire region of upstate New York named after them, or that the humble chicken soup would prove to have medicinal qualities? A Jewish doctor, indeed!

If necessity is the mother of invention, Jewish tradition is a matriarch. The perennially popular matzo ball soup is a modified dumpling soup suitable for Passover, connecting it with the exodus from Egypt and the commandment to observe *hag hamatzot*, a "holiday of matzos," every spring to commemorate liberation from slavery. Laurie Koehler shares her recipe handed down from her grandmother, who "immigrated" from Milwaukee to Seattle in 1892. Each year she takes out the special matzo ball soup pot, fills it with the ingredients, and simmers it overnight in the tradition that's been kept alive for several generations.

Chulent (also "cholent"), or *hamin* (derived from the Hebrew word for "hot") in Sephardic and Israeli lingo, is the soul food of Jewish kitchens. This one-pot meal of meat, beans, vegetables, and sometimes hard boiled eggs allegedly dates back to ancient times, when Jews would bury the meal in a pot under embers to have a hot lunch on Shabbat, when cooking is forbidden. Berdine Bender remembers how her mother set it up before Shabbat, leaving it to cook in a wood stove or, later, in a heated oven, until the family returned from Shabbat morning services.

These comfort meals are accompanied by the spirits of our ancestors. Linda Morgan, nowadays her family's "chicken soup maven," writes Grandma Shirley's Chicken Soup that she inherited from her grandmother. Though it may seem as though she prepares her Jewish penicillin alone, she knows the truth: her grandmother is there with her at the stove as she prepares.

Rivy Poupko Kletenik's Baal Shem Tov Borscht, a second-night Passover Seder tradition, was always paired with her father's story of the "Escape from Velizhe," when the Poupko family escaped the Soviet Union under the direst of circumstances. Because of borscht, he always began, the Russians won the revolution.
They don't know why the soup is named for the Hassidic master, known as the "Besht" for short, but it surely is the "Besht" borscht outside of the Borscht Belt.

TIDBIT:
At the 2008 International Federation of Competitive Eaters, Joey Chestnut ate 78 matzo balls in eight minutes. Second place went to Pat Bertoletti, who ate 76 balls in eight minutes. The third-place finisher consumed a mere 40 matzo balls.

TIDBIT:

The Borscht Belt refers to the region of summer resorts, hotels, camps, and bungalows in the Catskills, New York, popular among Jews in the 1940s, 50s, and 60s. Borscht Belt humor, the self-deprecating comedy popularized by comedians like Rodney Dangerfield and Woody Allen, was born here. Example: "My doctor said I was in terrible shape. I told him, 'I want a second opinion.' He said, 'All right, you're ugly too!'"

JEWISH PENICILLIN TO THE BORSCHT BELT

BAAL SHEM TOV'S BORSCHT

Rivy Poupko Kletenik

"This is our family's traditional soup served at our Second Seder. We are not clear why my mother called it the Baal Shem Tov's Borscht – perhaps it was the other-worldly mystical quality of this sublime elixir that demanded a name with a corresponding holiness. It was at our Second Seder too, over bowls of borscht, that my father would tell the story of 'Escape from Velizhe'; how the Poupko family stole out of the former Soviet Union, despite imminent internment in Siberia and house arrest. It was a tale that always began with how it was because of borscht that the Russians won the Revolution. Of course, borscht-eating Russians were fighting on both sides of that revolution."

Serves 12

5 pounds beets, peeled and sliced
2 onions, peeled but kept whole
2 pounds flanken (beef short ribs)
1 package beef marrow bones
1 package beef neck bones
Salt, to taste
Sugar, to taste
2 lemons, juiced

Place the beets, onions, flanken, marrow bones, and neck bones in a large pot. Add enough water to cover and bring the soup to a boil, then reduce to a simmer. Cook for 2 hours, skimming the foam that rises to the top as often as you like.

Allow the soup to cool. Remove the onions and bones.

Adjust the seasoning in order to get to a sweet and sour flavor by adding a few tablespoons of sugar and the lemon juice.

SWEET AND SOUR CABBAGE SOUP

Morrene Jacobson

Makes 8 hearty servings

2 pounds lean boneless beef, cut into 1-inch cubes
1 28-ounce can diced tomatoes, with their juice
1 cup tomato sauce
2 pounds green cabbage, shredded or thinly sliced
2 medium onions, sliced
1 teaspoon sour salt
2 teaspoons kosher salt
½ teaspoon pepper
3 tablespoons sugar
6 tablespoons raisins

Combine the beef and 2 quarts of water in a 10-quart soup pot. Bring to a boil and skim off the foam that rises to the top. Add the tomatoes and juice, tomato sauce, cabbage, onions, sour salt, kosher salt, pepper, and sugar. Bring the soup back to a boil, stirring occasionally. Cover and simmer for 3 hours.

Add the raisins and simmer the soup with the lid askew for 20 minutes. Adjust the seasoning, if necessary.

TIPS & TRICKS:

- ❖ Sour salt is citric acid, which you may find in the spice section at the grocery store or in the kosher section.
- ❖ After the soup has simmered for 3 hours, I like to take the beef out and shred it before returning it to the pot. Or, you can leave the cubes in, if you prefer.

"When we were growing up, Friday night dinner attendees always included my parents, Florence and Ben Maslan, the six of us kids, and our maternal grandparents, Abe and Anna Silver. Sometimes there would be uncles, aunts, cousins, or friends from school, AZA, BBG, or Young Judea. Occasionally, my father would bring home guests, expected or unexpected, like the Lieutenant Governor of California or the Lord Mayor of Dublin. Sometimes it was the speaker or entertainer at the upcoming JNF or Israel Bonds dinner. Attendance at our Shabbat dinners grew to a standard of 25 to 30 guests every week. Never flustered by the large crowd, my mother would always say, 'No problem, I will throw some more water in the soup.'

"It might have been chicken soup, sometimes with rice, or sometimes with noodles of different widths, or during the holidays, simmering matzo balls. Besides chicken soup, there was usually a vegetable soup, usually beef-based, sometime with marrow. Leftover soup always went into the freezer and then was added to the next batch. We referred to the new product as 'Thousand Year Soup.'"

~ Ruth Sassoon

GRANDMA SHIRLEY'S CHICKEN SOUP

Linda Morgan

"Shirley Teitelbaum, my grandmother (my mother Frances Rogers' mother) was a widely respected cook, who gleaned her recipes and culinary ability from the 'old country.' While we cherished her famed cakes and cookies, I knew it was the 'Jewish mother' basic I wanted to master: Chicken Soup. So I invited her to my home one day many years ago, where I watched and learned.

"I hear her voice – even today – when I prepare this soup: 'Leave the celery leaves on; they add some bitterness to the flavor.' 'If you put a beef bone in, it will make the soup richer.' 'Always add the salt later.' 'Be sure to put the parsley in last of all.' And more: 'Kosher chicken has more flavor.' 'The onion should go in ½ hour from the start.' 'When the soup boils, skim off the foam...the soup should be clear.'

"My grandmother made this soup for every Jewish holiday, for Shabbat dinners, for her children, grandchildren, and great-grandchildren, should they need some Jewish penicillin. She added homemade pesachdik noodles for the Seder, kreplach for the holidays, and matzo balls just for fun. These days, I am the family chicken soup maven. And while it may look to others as if this is a solitary endeavor, I know the truth. I am chopping, boiling, skimming, and salting with Grandma Shirley. And that's a very good thing."

Serves 6

One whole chicken, cut into pieces
1 beef bone, rinsed
1 parsnip, peeled and halved
1/8 teaspoon black peppercorns
3 stalks celery (leaves on), chopped in 1/2-inch pieces
3 to 4 carrots, peeled and cut into thirds
1 clove garlic, halved
1 onion, halved
1/4 cup parsley, chopped
Salt

Wash the chicken and place in the pot. Add the beef bone and enough water so the chicken is just covered (about 8 cups). Bring the soup to a boil on high heat, skimming the foam continuously, so the soup is clear. Reduce the temperature to simmer and cover the pot.

Add the parsnip and peppercorns. Cover and simmer for 10 minutes. Add the celery, carrots, garlic, and onions. Simmer for about 90 minutes, add salt to taste, and then add the parsley. Simmer for another 30 minutes.

Strain the soup through a colander into a bowl large enough to hold the broth. Return the broth to the pot. Remove the bones and skin from the chicken and cut the chicken into pieces. Return just the chicken, carrots, and celery to the broth or leave the soup as a broth.

TIPS & TRICKS:

- For a Hungarian touch (from my mother-in-law, Edith Morgan): Add ¼ teaspoon of paprika and 1 green pepper (halved and seeded) to the broth at the same time as the celery, carrots, garlic, and onions.

KREPLACH

Lois Kaplan Glickman

Makes about 17 kreplach

Dough:
1½ cups flour
½ teaspoon baking powder
3 eggs
2 tablespoons water

Put the flour, baking powder, eggs, and water in a food processor and mix until well blended. Knead the dough, using additional flour if needed, until it is a good consistency for rolling out.

Filling:
½ yellow onion, diced
4 to 5 slices leftover roast beef or brisket, cut into ¼-inch cubes
1 egg, beaten

Sauté the onions, then combine with the meat, and grind in a food processor. Add the egg and mix completely.

Roll out the dough on a floured board, as you would for pie crust dough. Use a large biscuit cutter (about 2½-inches in diameter) to cut circles of dough.

Put 1 teaspoon of the filling in the center of each dough-circle. Fold the edges of the dough in toward the center until they overlap, pinching and crimping them together in the middle.

Arrange the kreplach in a single layer on a baking sheet and freeze for several hours. Then put them in freezer bags and store in the freezer until needed.

Bring a pot of chicken soup to a boil. Drop the kreplach into the soup and simmer for 30 to 45 minutes.

TIPS & TRICKS:

- This recipe makes enough dough for about 17 kreplach, but the filling is enough for 3 times that number. It is easier to handle and process the dough in the amounts given above.

KNEIDLACH (MATZO BALLS)

Natalie Malin

"This was my grandmother, Lena Greenberg Thomas', recipe. She was a great cook! I remember watching her, fascinated, while she made bagels, long before they were popular. She lived in Seattle, but her ancestors were originally from Germany and lived in a German colony in Courland, Latvia. There, they spoke 'High German' instead of Yiddish. My wonderful aunt, Dorothy Thomas Kraft, watched her prepare the traditional dishes, and carefully measured out the ingredients. Here is Dorothy's recipe for Kneidlach."

Makes 8 kneidlach

4 eggs
½ cup cold water (can use club soda instead)
⅓ cup oil or melted shortening
1 tablespoon plus 1 teaspoon salt
Dash of pepper
1 cup matzo meal

Beat the eggs and then add the water, oil, 1 teaspoon of the salt, and pepper. Mix well. Add the matzo meal and stir thoroughly. Refrigerate 45 to 60 minutes. Form into balls. Bring 1½ quarts water to a boil and add the remaining tablespoon of salt. Drop the balls into the water, cover, and boil softly for 30 to 40 minutes.

OUR MATZO BALL SOUP

Laurie Koehler

"My grandmother, Henriette Levinson Hirshberg Nathan Block, moved to Seattle from Milwaukee in 1892. Her family lived north of Green Lake, and her parents were founding members of Temple De Hirsch Sinai. This recipe has been enjoyed by our family for generations. Every holiday we pull out the special pot that is dedicated to our matzo ball soup, fill it with all the rich ingredients, and simmer it overnight. It is always delicious, but guess what? There is absolutely no chicken in it."

Serves 12

4 veal bones
4 beef marrow bones
1 lamb shank
1 pint fresh beef liver
1 package of oxtails
3 onions
3 stalks celery, cut into 3-inch pieces
3 carrots, peeled and cut into 1-inch pieces
1 turnip, quartered
1 parsnip, quartered
1 28-ounce can whole tomatoes, with their juices
1 tablespoon sugar
½ bunch parsley, chopped
Salt and pepper, to taste

In an 8 to 10 quart pot, add the veal and beef bones, lamb shank, liver, oxtails, onions, celery, carrots, turnip, parsnip, tomatoes, and sugar. Fill the pot with water to 1 inch from the top. Bring the pot to a boil, then reduce the heat to simmer, and cook the soup 12 hours or overnight, adding the parsley in the last hour.

Cool the soup, then strain through a colander into a bowl large enough to hold the broth, and discard the rest. Refrigerate the broth for several hours.

When ready to serve, skim off any fat that has hardened and reheat the broth, adding your favorite matzo balls, and seasoning with salt and pepper. The recipe I use is right off the matzo ball soup box.

TONY'S GAZPACHO

Tony Wartnik

Serves 4 to 6

1 large clove garlic, halved
3 cups tomato, peeled, seeded, and finely chopped
1 cucumber, peeled, seeded, and chopped
4 tablespoons green pepper. minced
½ cup sweet onion, chopped
2 tablespoons olive oil
2 teaspoons lemon juice
1 teaspoon salt
¼ teaspoon pepper
Dash of Tabasco sauce
1 cup tomato juice, chilled
¼ cup parsley, chopped
Avocado, chopped, as a garnish
Black olives, as a garnish
Salsa, as a garnish

Rub a mixing bowl with the garlic, then add the tomatoes, cucumber, green pepper, onion, olive oil, lemon juice, salt, pepper, Tabasco sauce, tomato juice, and parsley. Let the mixture chill for at least 4 hours. Garnish with the chopped avocado, black olives, and salsa.

GAZPACHO

Barbara Wolf

"This recipe was given to me by Gladys Rubinstein – a wonderful cook and an especially wonderful woman."

Serves 6

4 large tomatoes, peeled, seeded, and coarsely chopped
1 medium onion, coarsely chopped, plus additional as a garnish
1 large cucumber, peeled, and sliced, plus additional as a garnish
1 red pepper, seeded, and chopped, plus additional as a garnish
¼ jalapeno pepper, seeded, and chopped, plus additional as a garnish
1 clove garlic, minced
2 cups tomato juice
⅓ cup tomato purée
1 tablespoon olive oil
2 tablespoons red wine vinegar
½ teaspoon ground cumin
1 tablespoon lemon juice
1 teaspoon sugar
Dash of Tabasco sauce
Dash of Worcestershire sauce
Black pepper, to taste

Marinate the tomatoes, onion, cucumber, red pepper, jalapeno, and garlic in the tomato juice for 2 hours.

In a blender, purée the marinated vegetables with the tomato purée, olive oil, red wine vinegar, cumin, lemon juice, sugar, Tabasco sauce, Worcestershire sauce, and pepper. Make some ice cubes with the mixture to float in each serving.

Chill the gazpacho for several hours and serve cold with the chopped onion, cucumber, and peppers on the side.

TIPS & TRICKS:

- Canned tomatoes may be substituted for some of the fresh tomatoes.
- Try serving the soup with a dollop of sour cream, some chopped avocado, and coarsely chopped parsley as garnish.

BEEF BARLEY SOUP

Bobbi Bridge

"Bob's favorite soup is this beef barley soup. When we were first married, not knowing too much about cooking, I tried to make him this recipe. He complained there was not enough barley in it, so I tried again. That time I had a huge pot of barley, but no soup. The next time time, I made it just right. This recipe is like the baby bear's porridge – not too hot and not too cold – or in this case not too much barley and not too little – but just right. You can add or subtract as you like."

3 tablespoons olive oil
5 pounds beef short ribs
3½ quarts water
⅞ cup barley
1 onion, chopped
1 tablespoon salt
2 bay leaves
1 clove, whole
1 peppercorn
1 allspice, whole
1 cup celery, diced
1 cup carrots, diced
1 cup potatoes, diced
1 rutabaga, quartered (optional)
1 parsnip, quartered (optional)

In a Dutch oven, heat the oil over medium-high heat and brown the short ribs on all sides. In a large cooking pot, add the short ribs, water, barley, onion, salt, bay leaves, clove, peppercorn, and allspice. Cover, bring to a boil, then reduce the heat and simmer for 2 hours. Add the celery, carrots, potatoes, rutabaga, and parsnip; cover and simmer for 1 hour longer. Stir occasionally and be sure to watch the soup as it simmers, as it can easily burn or stick to the bottom.

Before serving, remove the bones, bay leaves, cloves, peppercorn, allspice, rutabaga, and parsnip. Chop the meat very coarsely, removing as much fat as possible.

MUSHROOM AND BARLEY SOUP

Joy Paltiel

"Warm food...warm memories. My mother was a strict follower of Jewish laws. This meant that she did her Shabbat cooking very early Friday morning before going to work. On those days, it was not unusual for my sister and me to wake up to the fabulous smells of chicken, fish, or even chulent. My mother would plead with us to taste her cooking and then ask, 'Does it need more salt?' We would protest loudly, claiming it was too early in the morning, but eventually we would give in. She would cover the stove burners with a well-worn sheet of tin she called a 'blech' and place the pot of food on the tin so that when she got home from work, she would turn on the burners to a low heat and keep the food warm from Friday night to Saturday evening, thus assuring a warm Saturday afternoon meal. I really loved it when she made this mushroom barley soup. I thought of it as the breakfast of champions. It is delicious, easy to make, hearty, and made with ingredients I am likely to have in the house or can easily get at any local grocery store."

Serves 4

5½ cups beef broth
⅔ cup quick-cooking barley
½ cup onion, chopped
2 cloves garlic, minced
1 teaspoon dried basil, crushed
½ teaspoon Worcestershire sauce
⅛ teaspoon pepper
2 cups mushrooms, sliced
½ cup carrots, shredded
2 tablespoons cornstarch
2 tablespoons water
1 tablespoon parsley, chopped

In a large soup pot, add the beef broth, barley, onion, garlic, basil, Worcestershire sauce, and pepper. Cover and simmer for 10 minutes, until the barley is tender. Stir in the mushrooms and carrots and simmer for an additional 5 minutes.

In a small bowl, combine the cornstarch and water and add that mixture to the soup. Cook and stir until slightly thickened and bubbly. Cook 2 more minutes, sprinkle with the parsley, and serve.

WINTER BARLEY SOUP

Faye Sarkowsky

Makes 8 servings

2 tablespoons olive oil
2½ pounds lamb stew meat, cut in 1½-inch chunks
6 cups hot water
½ cup barley
2 medium onions, sliced and divided
2 tablespoons parsley, chopped
2 teaspoons salt
¼ teaspoon pepper
1 bay leaf
1½ cups celery, chopped
1½ cups carrots, sliced
½ green pepper, chopped (optional)
¼ teaspoon thyme leaves

Heat the oil in a Dutch oven. Add the lamb and brown it on all sides over medium-high heat. Add the water, barley, ½ of the onions, parsley, salt, pepper, and bay leaf. Cover and simmer over low to medium heat for about 1½ hours.

Stir in the remaining onion, celery, carrots, green pepper, and thyme. Bring the soup to a simmer and cook uncovered for 30 minutes, until the meat is tender. Season to taste with salt and pepper and remove the bay leaf before serving.

CURRIED PEANUT – PUMPKIN SOUP

Goldie Tobin

Serves 6 to 8

Olive oil
1 onion, chopped
2 cloves garlic, minced
7/8 teaspoon curry powder (or 3/4 teaspoon for milder taste)
1/4 teaspoon cayenne pepper
1 28-ounce can pumpkin purée
1/2 cup smooth peanut butter
6 ounces apple juice from concentrate
3 14-ounce cans low sodium chicken broth (such as Swanson's)
Plain yogurt, as a garnish

Coat the bottom of a 5 to 6-quart pot with the olive oil. Heat over medium heat and add the onion, garlic, curry powder, and cayenne pepper, and sauté for 5 to 8 minutes. Add the pumpkin purée, peanut butter, apple juice, and chicken broth. Bring to a boil, then reduce heat, and simmer for 25 minutes. Cool slightly then purée with a food processor or hand blender.

Serve with a spoonful of yogurt in the center of each bowl.

TIPS & TRICKS:

- If the soup is too thick, add more chicken broth until the consistency is to your liking.

PASTA E FAGIOLI

Barbara Sulman

6 servings

2 cups white beans, dried
2 tablespoons olive oil
1 medium onion, chopped
2 carrots, peeled and chopped
2 celery stalks, chopped
4 cloves garlic, minced
8 cups chicken broth or water
1 14-ounce can chopped tomatoes, with the juice
Salt and pepper, to taste
2 tablespoons fresh thyme or 1 teaspoon dried thyme
½ head green cabbage, chopped
½ cup dried pasta shells, cooked
Parmesan cheese, grated, as a garnish

Pick through the beans and discard any misshapen beans or stones.

Rinse the beans, drain, and place in sauce pan with enough water to cover and bring to a boil. Boil for 2 minutes, remove from heat, cover, let stand for 1 hour, then drain.

In a soup pot, heat the olive oil, then add the onion, carrots, celery, and garlic and sauté, stirring until the vegetables soften.

Add the chicken broth, drained beans, tomatoes, salt, pepper, and thyme. Bring to a boil, then add the cabbage. Cover, reduce heat to low, and simmer until the beans are tender, approximately 1 hour.

To give the soup more body, remove three cups of the soup and cool. Purée in a blender and return to the soup pot.

Add the pasta and reheat. Serve the soup warm with Parmesan cheese as a garnish.

CHULENT

Berdine Bender

"Growing up, my mother's chulent recipe was a favorite Shabbos Friday night or Saturday meal for our whole family. Traditionally, chulent would be set up to cook prior to the start of Shabbos and left to cook in a wood stove with smoldering coals or, more recently, in a preheated oven that remained unopened until the family returned from Saturday morning services. One would have a warm, delicious meal that needed no tending over Shabbos.

"As the years passed, and I had two children of my own, my mother would always please her grandchildren with this same Shabbos delicacy. Sadly, as she aged and had several strokes, she lost her ability to remember moment to moment, but always retained her social graces and desire to be the 'balabust' to her children and grandchildren. Though she had long lost the facility to remember the way to cook even this simple recipe, she would repeatedly ask my family, one by one, 'Tell me, do you like chulent?' Even though she could no longer make the recipe, she still warmed our hearts with the thought of this tasty meal and with the warmth and grace with which she posed this question."

Serves 6 to 8

1 chicken, cut up
5 potatoes, peeled and quartered
½ pound dried lima beans
2 tablespoons cinnamon
Salt to taste

Preheat the oven to 350°.

Put the chicken pieces in a large ovenproof pot. Fill the pot with enough water to just cover the chicken. Bring to a boil and skim the foam off the top.

Add the potatoes, beans, salt, and cinnamon to the chicken.

Place the pot, uncovered, into the preheated oven and bake until most of the water has disappeared and the chicken and potatoes are brown, at least 3 to 4 hours.

CHICKEN STEW

Ruthie Winston

"I love this chicken recipe that was given to me by one of my Sephardic friends. It's comfort food in a pot."

Serves 6

1 fryer chicken, cut into pieces
2 tablespoons oil
2 medium onions, sliced
1 28-ounce can tomatoes with juice
½ lemon, juiced
1 teaspoon sugar
Salt and pepper to taste
4 medium potatoes, quartered

Brown the chicken lightly in the oil.

Line a greased Dutch oven with the sliced onions and place the chicken over the onions.

In a separate bowl, mix the tomatoes with lemon juice, sugar, and salt and pepper to taste. Pour this mixture over the chicken. Cover and let simmer for 30 minutes.

Add the potatoes, cover the Dutch oven, and cook for 45 to 60 minutes until the potatoes are tender and the chicken is done.

AFRICAN PEANUT STEW

Terry Bloom

"This recipe is a favorite of my grandkids at Halloween. I also like it for an informal winter dinner with friends. It is nice as an entrée when vegetarians are present."

Serves 8

1 tablespoon olive oil
1 medium red onion, chopped
1 stalk celery, chopped
½ cup carrot, chopped
3 cloves garlic, peeled and minced
2 tablespoons fresh ginger, peeled, and minced
1 tablespoon curry powder
1 14-ounce can fire-roasted tomatoes, with their juices
1 cup vegetable broth
1 large sweet potato, diced
¼ cup creamy peanut butter
1 pound protein: cooked, shredded chicken; tofu; or edamame (optional)
¼ cup fresh cilantro, chopped
5 ounces baby spinach
½ teaspoon salt, or to taste
Black pepper, to taste
Brown rice, cooked
½ cup chopped peanuts, as a garnish

In a large soup pot, sauté the onion, celery, and carrot in olive oil for about 5 minutes. Add the garlic, ginger, and curry powder, and sauté until fragrant. Do not brown the garlic.

Add the tomatoes and cook uncovered for about 3 to 5 minutes, reducing the liquid slightly. Add the vegetable broth and sweet potatoes, and bring the mixture to a boil. Reduce the heat to low and simmer the stew for about 10 minutes. Add the peanut butter and the protein, if desired. Stir until well mixed.

Continue to simmer the stew, covered, for about 45 minutes. Stir in the cilantro and the spinach. Season to taste with salt and pepper. Serve over the brown rice and garnish with the chopped peanuts.

LENTIL STEW

Morrene Jacobson

Makes 6 hearty servings

2 tablespoons olive oil
2 cups yellow onion, diced
2 cups carrots, diced
1 tablespoon garlic, minced
2 teaspoons ground cumin
1 cup dried lentils, rinsed
4 cups chicken broth
1 28-ounce can diced tomatoes, with their juice
1 tablespoon brown sugar
1 3-inch cinnamon stick
½ cup barley
1 pound extra firm tofu, rinsed and cut into ½-inch cubes
½ cup Italian parsley, chopped
Salt and pepper, to taste

Heat the oil in a large, heavy pot. Cook the onions and carrots, stirring occasionally, for 8 minutes. Add the garlic and cook for 2 minutes. Add the cumin and cook, stirring, for 1 minute.

Stir in the lentils, broth, tomatoes with their juice, brown sugar, and cinnamon stick. Bring to a boil then reduce the heat and simmer, with the pot partially covered, for 5 minutes. Add the barley and simmer, with the pot partially covered, for 45 minutes, stirring occasionally. Gently stir in the tofu during the last 5 minutes.

Add the parsley, and season to taste with salt and pepper. Simmer for a few minutes longer to let the flavors blend. Remove the cinnamon stick before serving.

TIPS & TRICKS:

❖ One large onion should yield 2 cups of onion and 4 large carrots should give you the 2 cups of carrots.

TAGINE WITH CARROTS, POTATOES, AND OLIVES

Dana Wootton

"At the age of 16, I announced to my mother that I was no longer eating meat. Rather than chastise me, she started to re-imagine what dinner could look like at our house. She began to experiment more in the kitchen, bringing in the food of other cultures. Suddenly, I was exposed to a whole new world of tastes and textures, and food was never the same old boring thing for me again. I learned the creative spark from my mom, and I also learned that food brings joy to so many different people in our lives. This recipe may look overwhelming, but many of the ingredients are spices and really, it just a bunch of chopping and letting the deliciousness happen on its own."

Serves 4

2/3 cup plain whole milk yogurt
1/2 to 3/4 teaspoon curry powder
Olive oil
1 large onion, diced
Pinch of salt
2 teaspoons ground cumin
1 teaspoon ground coriander
1/2 teaspoon tumeric
1/2 teaspoon paprika
Large pinch of cayenne pepper
Pinch of saffron threads
2 to 3 large carrots, cut into 1/4-inch slices
3 medium red potatoes, cut into 1-inch pieces
1 red pepper, seeded and cut into 1-inch pieces
1 yellow pepper, seeded and cut into 1-inch pieces
1 14-ounce can diced tomatoes
1 cup water
1 14-ounce can chickpeas, drained
1/3 cup kalamata olives, coarsely chopped
10 large prunes, coarsely chopped
1/4 cup parsley, chopped

Mix the yogurt and curry powder in a bowl. Cover and chill.

Heat a large Dutch oven over medium heat. Add just enough olive oil to coat the bottom and then add the onions and a large pinch of salt. Sauté until the onion starts to soften, but not brown. Add the salt, cumin, coriander, turmeric, paprika, cayenne pepper, and saffron, and stir to coat the onions well. Add the potatoes and carrots and mix well.

Add the red and yellow peppers, tomatoes, and water. Stir, increase the heat, and bring the mixture to a boil. Cover and lower the heat to medium-low. Cook for 10 minutes and then add the chickpeas, olives, and prunes. Cover again and cook until the vegetables are tender, about another 15 minutes. About 5 minutes before serving, add the parsley. Serve with a dollop of the curried yogurt on top.

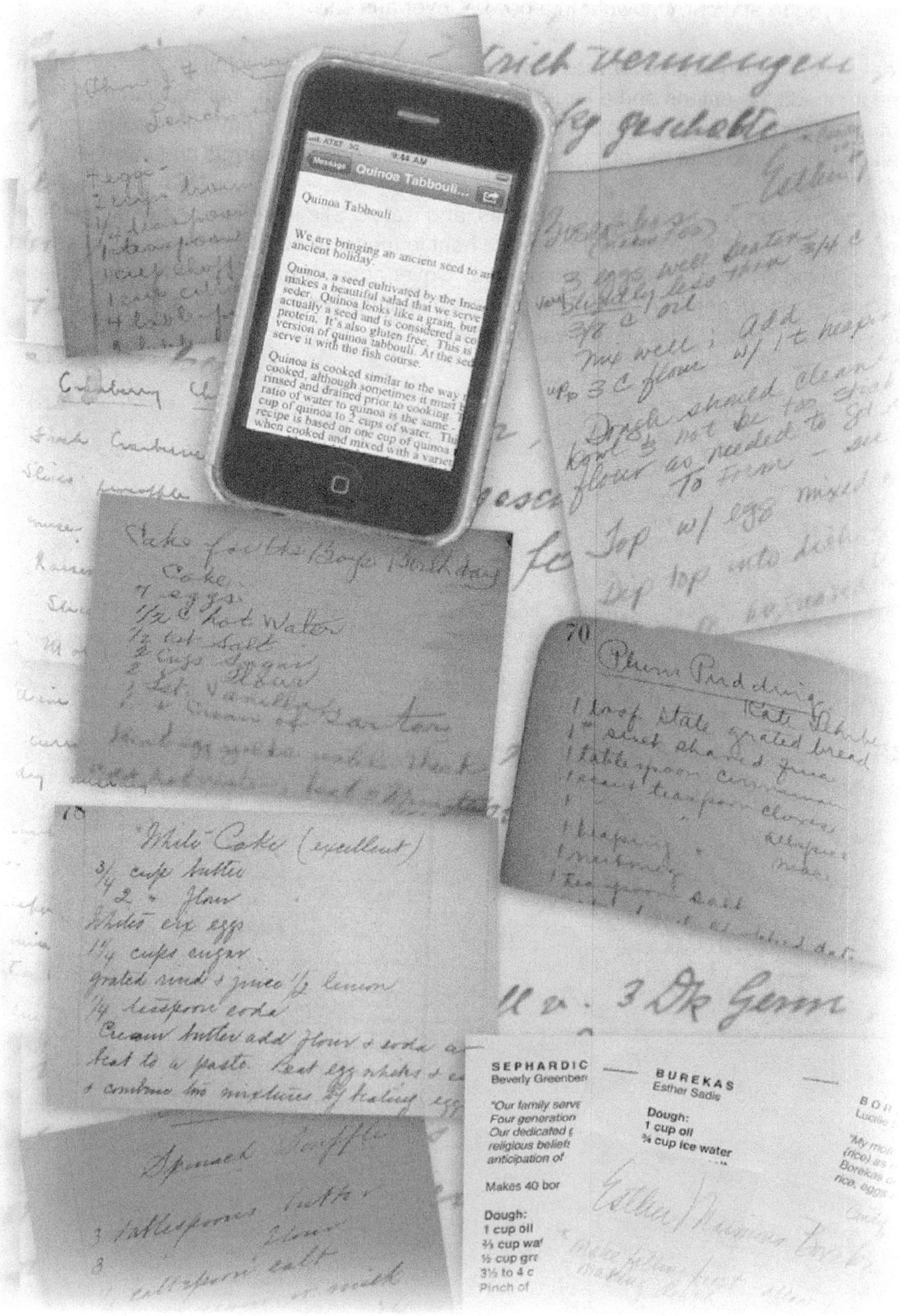
Quinoa Tabbouli...
Quinoa Tabbouli
SEPHARDIC
BUREKAS
Esther Sadie
Dough:
1 cup oil
¾ cup ice water
"White Cake (excellent)
Plum Pudding

Prasas to Cabbage

When we think of Jewish food, vegetables aren't exactly the first thing to come to mind. Corned beef on rye smeared with spicy mustard, maybe, or a melt-in-your-mouth matzo ball, sweet challah dipped in salt, roast chicken, a crunchy biscocho or a boreka bulging with potato and cheese. Jewish vegetarians, although making strong headway, frequently encounter stunned responses to their dietary values. "But do you eat fish?" is assuredly the next question.

Vegetarians aside, vegetables – alone or combined with meat – not only enhance every traditional Jewish dish, but they also pack historical and spiritual significance. They make an appearance at every festival: At Passover, we taste parsley, lettuce, or celery to hearken back to our ancestral days of slavery; on Hanukkah we fry potatoes in oil to remember the existence of miracles; on Sukkot we feast on the autumn harvest. Seattle's Sephardic Jews from Rhodes and Turkey incorporate leeks into both Rosh Hashanah and Passover meals. According to Eugene and Esther Normand, the leek is highly regarded by Mediterranean people and included in the *Yehi Ratzones*, a mini-Seder held during the Rosh Hashanah meal. Celery root, okra, eggplant and tomatoes also factor strongly into Sephardic, Israeli, and Middle Eastern Jewish culinary customs.

While a variety of vegetables were available to Sephardic Jews in warmer climates, Ashkenazi Jews in Eastern Europe assimilated root vegetables and cabbage. This region can be thanked for the legacy of sauerkraut, which Dorothy Becker nostalgically praises via her memories of Hinda August's beloved old country recipe, made with a mallet in her hand and a *schmata* over the crock.

The Pacific Northwest adds an exciting angle. The abundance of local farm initiatives and the rise of urban gardening in Seattle will no doubt influence our community's cooking. Already we have Goldie Tobin's Marinated Sweet Walla Walla Onions. Healthy, local recipes in an age of health- and environmental-consciousness bring vegetables the attention they deserve and contribute to the continual innovation upon tradition.

TIDBIT:

An American traveling through Russia asked a peasant why the locals expressed so much anti-Semitism. The peasant answered, "It is because the Jews have a secret vegetable they eat so they don't become alcoholics like the rest of us. And they refuse to share that vegetable with anyone else."

Amy Fine Collins. "Jewish Like Me." *Vanity Fair* (2008).

PRASAS TO CABBAGE

HINDA'S CABBAGE (SAUERKRAUT)

Dorothy Becker

"This recipe of Hinda August's was in the Bikur Cholim newsletter in 1988. Hinda was born in Ostrow, Poland in 1895. During World War I, she was a frontline nurse and moved to Seattle to join her husband in 1921. She and her husband started a business of making garlic dill pickles which they shipped to Alaska, earning 50 cents a barrel. Hinda's sauerkraut was also famous and represents a true 'old country' family-cherished recipe. It can be made in a gallon crock the old fashioned way with a cutter, a wooden mallet and a 'schmata.'"

Makes 1 to 2 quarts

3 to 4 heads green cabbage
1/3 cup table salt
Caraway seeds and carrot slivers, optional

Shred or cut the cabbage into medium to coarse sized pieces. Pack in layers in a crock, a layer of cabbage then a teaspoon of salt sprinkled over. After the last salt addition, mash the cabbage down with a mallet until some liquid appears. Continue until all the cabbage is used. If you desire to use the caraway seeds and the carrots, layer them along with the cabbage. You should have quite a bit of liquid in the crock, and it should cover the cabbage. Be sure to leave room at the top of the crock. To be sure the cabbage remains submerged, put a small plate over the cabbage and weigh it down with a small, clean rock placed in a small plastic bowl.

Cover the crock with a schmata (tea towel) and secure it with a string. Place the crock in a cool place like an unheated garage. Every few days, "burp" the crock by pressing down on the saucer; bubbles will appear. Remove any scum and wash the saucer occasionally. If the sauerkraut seems dry, add a little warm water. Cover the crock again. Repeat this process every few days.

In about 10 days, the sauerkraut will taste wonderful. At that point you can put it in jars and keep it in the refrigerator.

BECKY'S CARROT SOUFFLE

Becky Benaroya

"A dear friend and neighbor, Bess Agin, gave me this recipe over 50 years ago when we lived in Cleveland for a short time. She was a wonderful cook. I had never tasted anything like this, and I still haven't anywhere. I always serve it with our Thanksgiving meal."

Serves 12

3 cups all-purpose flour
1½ teaspoons baking soda
1½ teaspoons baking powder
1½ teaspoons cinnamon
¾ teaspoon nutmeg
3 cups shortening, creamed
1½ cups brown sugar
6 eggs, separated
4½ cups carrots, grated
3 tablespoons lemon juice
3 tablespoons water

Preheat the oven to 350°. Grease a 9-inch Bundt pan well.

Combine the flour, baking soda, baking powder, cinnamon, and nutmeg in a bowl.

In an electric mixer, cream the shortening and mix in the sugar and egg yolks. Stir in the carrots then add the flour mixture. Add the lemon juice and water and mix until just combined.

Beat the egg whites until stiff peaks form. With a rubber spatula, fold the egg whites into the carrot mixture. Spoon into the prepared pan and smooth the top. Bake for 45 minutes to 1 hour, or until a toothpick comes out clean.

TIPS & TRICKS:

- This can be made in a 9x13-inch glass dish if you prefer, but it won't take quite as much time to cook.
- I use "I Can't Believe It's Not Butter" instead of traditional shortening.

APIO (CELERY ROOT)

Lilly DeJaen

"Apio can be used as a side dish, a salad or an appetizer. It is both sweet and sour. I always serve it cold for Passover. The flavor improves with standing, so prepare it ahead."

Makes 2 to 3 cups

1 large or 2 medium celery root bulbs, peeled, cut in quarters
2 carrots, peeled and sliced diagonally
2 or 3 celery stalks, sliced diagonally
2 tablespoons oil
2 tablespoons sugar (or to taste)
1 teaspoon salt
2 lemons, juiced (or to taste)

Slice the peeled celery root quarters into ¼-inch pieces.

In a saucepan, add the oil, sugar, salt, lemon juice and enough water to cover the vegetables, which you will add later. Bring to a boil. Lower heat to medium and add the celery root and carrots. Cook until tender. Just before celery root and carrots finish cooking, add the sliced celery stalks and cook until the vegetables are tender, but not falling apart. If needed add a little more water.

FRIEDALA'S RED CABBAGE

Frieda Sondland

Friedala's Red Cabbage recipe was given to Frieda by her mother, Lina Piepsch, who got it from her Polish mother.

Serves 8 to 10

1 medium size red cabbage
⅓ cup dark raisins
½ cup lemon juice
2 to 3 Granny Smith apples, unpeeled and diced into chunks
2 to 3 cups water

Combine the cabbage, raisins, lemon juice, apples, and water in a large pot and simmer for 2 to 3 hours, until all ingredients are soft and well-blended. If all the water evaporates, add more as needed.

FRIED LEEK PATTIES (PRASAFUCHIS)

Esther and Eugene Normand

"Leek, or prasa *as it is known in Ladino and many of the Balkan languages, is a vegetable highly esteemed by all Mediterranean people. This vegetable, which looks and smells like a large green onion, is widely used by Greeks, Italians, and others in salads and soups. The Sephardic Jews of the former Ottoman Empire prepare leek dishes which include prasafuchis (the unadulterated fried leek patty), kifteh de prasa (patty of leek and hamburger) and novya de prasa, (the white portion of the leek stuffed with hamburger). Prasa in some form is expected to be served on Rosh Hashanah, at which the Sephardim have a mini-Seder like service based on seven foods called the* Yehi Ratzones. *In our family, the favorite form is the pure prasafuchi, partly because of its wonderful taste, but also due to the extensive preparation that is required to make it.*

"Also, in a traditional Turkish Sephardic home, a Passover Seder table is not complete without prasafuchis. In Seattle, leeks are usually easy to obtain in the produce section of most supermarkets. But that isn't the case everywhere! We remember the Passover of 1972 which we call the Pesach of Bedikat Prasa *(Passover of the Searching for the Leek). In that year our family lived in Chicago, and our parents/in-laws, Sam and Lucy Maimon, came to visit and spend Passover with us. Passover is usually in April, but April in Chicago is not the same as April in Seattle: April in Chicago can mean snow and cold.*

"That year, the first Seder was actually on a Wednesday evening at the end of March, so the first forays into the grocery and vegetables stores began on Monday, but we had no luck. On Tuesday, Esther and her father, a former grocer (24th Avenue Market *on Yesler Way for more than 30 years) met with the same results. We thought that we were competing with the Greeks and Armenians who wanted leeks for part of their Easter meals, but it was really the terrible weather that kept out most of the leek shipments. Finally on Wednesday, with the snow coming down, Esther and her dad found four scrawny prasas, not much bigger than scallions, but still they were prasa. Esther's Mom, Lucy, an excellent cook the year round, knew what to do with them, as small as they were. She made them into enough prasafuchis for us to all enjoy as they were rationed out to cover both Seder meals.*

"At the Sephardic synagogue, we found out that most of the Sephardim in Chicago hadn't even tried to make prasa; it just wasn't available. However, they did tell us where the large vegetable market was located. We drove there on Sunday, but only a few merchants were at their stalls, and in Greek they told my father-in-law to come back on Monday morning. I did, returning via the elevated subway, and much to my amazement, I found as much prasa as I could ever want. The Greek dealer had been out of it for a week, but he had just received a large shipment from California, and I bought 8 bunches. It was beautiful prasa, and some of its distinctive aroma was left behind that day in an otherwise prosaic engineering office. My mother-in-law made both prasafuchis and kiftehs de prasa for the second days of Passover, which we enjoyed all the more while remembering the meager prasafuchis of the Seder nights the previous week."

Makes about ten 3-inch patties

3 to 4 large leeks, white and light green parts only
1 sheet matzo, slightly moistened
1 egg
½ teaspoon salt
Vegetable oil for frying

Cut off the roots and tough outer leaves of the leek and cut them into large pieces. Wash them well, changing the water several times, until all the dirt is removed.

Place the leeks in a large saucepan. Add just enough water to cover the leeks and boil until tender (approximately 45 minutes). The leeks will turn from bright green to a pea green. Drain well, squeeze out all the water, and cool.

Chop then process or grind (preferred) the leeks. Place the matzo, egg, and salt in a large mixing bowl. Add the leeks and mix thoroughly. If the mixture is not thick enough, use more matzo. Form into small patties. In a large fry pan over high heat, heat enough oil to come up ½-inch from the bottom of the pan. Fry the patties until golden.

"My recipe for Fritas de Prasas (leek patties) was passed down to me by my late beloved mother, Lisa Benaroya, and goes back to my great-grandmother, all of whom lived in Edirne, Turkey. This recipe is used every Rosh Hashanah and Pesach. It is well known and loved by Sephardim originating mostly from the Balkan countries.

"In our family, as in many others, leek patties are eaten in particular during part of a small Seder on the two nights of Rosh Hashanah. These are made parve. A blessing is recited in Hebrew, and/or in Ladino and/or English, for each of the items of the Seder (apple & honey/sugar, dates, spinach, pumpkin or zucchini, and fish.) This series of prayers are called Yehi Ratzones.

"For Pesach, my mother made the patties with meat, to be eaten as part of the meal and savored by all."

~ Judith Amiel

ROASTED CAULIFLOWER THE WAY WE LIKE IT

Brooke Benaroya Dickson

"We make this super-simple side all the time. It's great mixed into whole wheat pasta or as a side dish to accompany a favorite protein – pan-seared halibut, roast chicken or grilled, sliced steak."

Serves 6

1 head cauliflower, cut into florets
1 to 2 tablespoons olive oil
Salt and pepper
1 to 2 cloves garlic, minced (optional)
Several sprigs flat leaf parsley, chopped
1 to 2 lemons, juiced and zested
¼ cup almonds, pine nuts, or pistachios, toasted and chopped
Salt and pepper

Preheat the oven to 425°.

In a bowl, toss the cauliflower florets with the olive oil, salt, pepper, and garlic. Place in an oven-safe pan or baking dish large enough to hold the cauliflower in a single layer. Roast for about 15 minutes, checking and stirring once or twice to ensure even roasting.

When ready, transfer the cauliflower from the pan and into a large bowl. While still warm, toss it with the parsley, lemon juice, lemon zest, and toasted nuts.

Sprinkle with salt and pepper to taste and serve.

EGGPLANT PIE

Jack Richlen

Serves 6 to 8

1 eggplant, peeled and sliced into ¼-inch thick rounds
1 teaspoon to 1 tablespoon garlic (as you prefer), minced
1 tomato, sliced
1 red bell pepper, sliced vertically into ¼-inchx3-inch pieces
1 small onion, sliced in rounds
1 teaspoon oregano
1 to 2 tablespoons olive oil
4 to 6 ounces mozzarella or cheddar cheese
¼ cup Parmesan cheese, grated

Broil eggplant slices on both sides until lightly brown.

Preheat the oven to 350°.

Layer the eggplant slices in a pie plate. Sprinkle minced garlic evenly over the top. In layers, add tomato, pepper, and onion. Sprinkle the oregano evenly over the top. Drizzle olive oil over the entire pie.

Bake the pie for 25 minutes. Top with the mozzarella or cheddar cheese and sprinkle the Parmesan cheese. Bake 10 minutes more, until cheeses are melted.

TIPS & TRICKS:

- The eggplant pie makes a great potluck dish.
- The eggplant can also be fried. This helps remove extra moisture.

SIMPLY BRAISED ENDIVE

Brooke Benaroya Dickson

"Braising brings out the sweetness in endive, making it a great side dish."

Serves 6

8 to 10 Belgian endive
Salt and pepper
1 tablespoon olive oil
1 cup chicken or vegetable stock (approximate)
½ cup dry white wine

Preheat the oven to 400°.

Trim the root ends of the endive and remove the outer leaves if discolored. Cut the endive in half lengthwise, through the root, and season with salt and pepper.

Over medium heat, heat a fry pan and add the olive oil. Add the endive cut side down and sauté until golden brown. Using tongs, flip the endive to the cut side up and pour in the chicken stock and white wine. Cook the endive until tender, about 20 to 25 minutes, and serve.

TIPS & TRICKS:

- Either use a sauté pan that will hold the endive snugly in a single layer and go in the oven, or brown endive in batches and transfer to a baking dish that will hold it all.
- Fennel wedges can also be prepared this way.

OKRA
Beverly DeJaen

Serves 6 to 8

2 cloves garlic, thinly sliced
3 tablespoons tomato sauce
1 lemon, juiced
2 tablespoons oil
½ teaspoon sugar
½ teaspoon salt
½ cup water (if using fresh okra, use 1 cup water)
2 packages frozen okra (or 1 pound fresh, with tops and bottom tips trimmed)

Bring the garlic, tomato sauce, lemon juice, oil, sugar, salt, and water to a boil in a medium saucepan. Boil for 3 minutes then add the okra. Cover and simmer for 15 to 20 minutes. Make sure the okra does not fall apart. Serve hot.

TIPS & TRICKS:

❖ If desired, you can put the cooked okra into a pie dish and bake at 350° until the top is golden brown.

MARINATED WALLA WALLA SWEET ONIONS
Goldie Tobin

Serves 8

½ cup sugar
¾ cup white vinegar
½ cup water
1½ teaspoons dried dill
4 cups Walla Walla sweet onions, sliced
2 cups English cucumbers, sliced
Fresh dill, as a garnish

Bring the sugar, vinegar, water, and dill to a boil. Pour over the onions and cucumbers and refrigerate overnight. Sprinkle some fresh dill over the onions before serving. Serve cold.

MAMAW BRINIE'S SQUASH PIE

Laurie Rosenberg Rose

"My grandmother, Bertha Siegel Rubenstein, who was fondly referred to as Mamaw Brinie, was born in St. Louis, Missouri. When she was a teenager, her family moved to Dallas, Texas, where she met and married Sidney Rubenstein. Growing up in Dallas, my family shared countless hours at my grandparent's home. Spending time in Mamaw's kitchen preparing holiday meals are some of my fondest memories. I remember my great-grandmother, grandmother, and mother talking and laughing in Yiddish. Although I couldn't understand much of what they were saying, I cherished the moments of love, devotion, respect for Jewish traditions, family, and friends. There were many holidays spent at my grandparents' home with numerous aunts, uncles, cousins, extended family, and friends. These celebrations always included a meal at a long dining room table with card table extensions covered with beautiful tablecloths.

"When Mamaw turned 75 years old, we had a party for her. For her special birthday, we assembled a cookbook with some of our favorite recipes borrowed from Mamaw's recipe box. The following squash recipe was, and still is, one of my favorites."

Serves 6 to 8

6 yellow squash, coarsely chopped
1 stalk celery, chopped into 1-inch chunks
2 carrots, peeled and cut into 1-inch pieces
1 small onion, coarsely chopped
1 new potato, peeled and cut into quarters
1 bell pepper, top removed, seeded, and chopped into ½-inch pieces (can use a red pepper)
1 zucchini
¼ cup canola oil
1 egg
¾ cup matzo meal
Salt and pepper, to taste

Preheat the oven to 350°. Grease an 8x8-inch glass dish.

Boil the squash in a bit of water until tender, about 7 minutes. Drain and put into a large bowl.

Sauté the celery, carrots, onion, potato, pepper, and zucchini until tender and combine with the squash. Add the oil, egg, matzo meal, and seasonings to taste. Blend everything in a food processor until quite smooth and pour into the prepared baking dish. Bake for 45 to 60 minutes, until golden brown.

Old Country Kugels to Rhodesli Rice

Most food traditions have a signature starch. In the case of Jewish tradition, one dish of Ashkenazi heritage stands out in American Jewish cooking: *Kugel.*

Following the same trend that produced such time-honored Jewish creations as gefilte fish and chulent, kugel and latkes are of the hybrid variety, a cross-pollination of surrounding European culture and Jewish law subject to centuries of innovation. The kugel, as far as we can trace it back, emerged in medieval Germany, where it appeared as a sort of casserole made with grains or bread and sausage. Due to its round shape, it became identified as kugel – "ball" or "sphere" in German. The Jews adapted it by omitting the sausage and letting the stew-like composite cook overnight on top of the Shabbat chulent. Over time, Jews followed the suit of the larger culture, adding honey, spices, eggs, or cheese, and changing out the grains for noodles or potatoes. From the fifteenth century on, kugel emerged as a mainstay of Jewish cooking.

Perhaps mavens of yore considered themselves innovative foodies by innovating kugel with raisins, cheese, and spices. But what was once perhaps truly inventive is now a bastion of traditionalism. Both Rivy Poupko Kletenik and Sandy Glass reminisce about their favorite potato kugels brought over from Poland and Romania, respectively. Alice Siegal reminisces about being a child in the 1930s, when the aroma of her mother's dairy kugel would fill the air before coming out of the oven golden, shiny, and deliciously cheesy.

While no equivalent to the popular kugel is represented here from the Sephardic world, we are happy to share dishes that highlight the Middle Eastern and Mediterranean staples like lentils, rice, and beans. The strong tradition of learning Sephardic recipes at the feet of the masters comes through here, as in Esther Sadis's story of the hours she spent mastering the craft of her mother-in-law's lentils and the dying art of Sephardic cooking.

Like the kugel, the humble potato pancake, or the latke, derives from the utility and resources of the old world. The crispy, oily patties whose oniony smell permeates the air inside Jewish homes every winter in celebration of Chanukah, are prepared across cultures and are even the national dish of Belarus. American foodies play with the basic ingredients, coming up with creations like Wendy Lynne's gluten-free carrot-scallion latke and butternut squash latke.

TIDBIT:

Every year since 1946, select college campuses have held a humorous philosophical symposium to argue the merits of the *latke* versus the *hamentasch.* At the Great Latke-Hamentasch Debate, opponents have invoked metaphysics, Greek philosophy, Freudian psychoanalysis, literary criticism and environmental ethics to prove that one Jewish treat is better than the other.

"Latke-Hamentasch Debate." *Wikipedia.*

Some recipe stories conjure up American history, like Brenda Atkin's memory of her father purchasing wild rice from the Native Americans in Minnesota, and others forge new traditions, like Anne Masin's all-American comfort food, Four Cheese Rigatoni. Every dish, whether creamy, saucy, or crispy, has the same memory-rich effect of comfort food on the brain and stomach.

TIDBIT:

In South African slang, *kugel* refers to young Jewish women who shunned the traditional lifestyle of their elders and gravitated instead toward materialism and ostentation. The insult was coined in the 1980s and expanded to cover not only Jewish "princesses" but Greek, Italian, Lebanese, and so forth, as well. The term implies that the woman, like the noodle dish, is dressed up but underneath actually is very plain.

Sarah Britten, "The Art of the South African Insult".
"Kugel." *Wikipedia.*
Gil Marks. *Olive Trees and Honey.*

OLD COUNTRY KUGELS TO RHODESLI RICE

POTATO AND CARROT KUGEL

Rivy Kletenik

"This recipe was given to my mother by her dear friend, Rebbetzin Blanka Gross, who returned to Poland from America in the late 1930s to care for her ailing father. Though an American citizen, she was interned at Bergen Belsen after sending her daughter Ruthie on the Kindertransport to the United Kingdom. She survived the war and returned to Pittsburgh, where she raised her family. Her granddaughter married my first cousin! This kugel is a huge family favorite – an ultimate comfort food for sure!"

Serves 12 to 16

4 eggs, beaten
4 carrots, peeled
6 potatoes, peeled
3 tablespoons canola oil
1 teaspoon salt

Preheat the oven to 350°. Grease or spray a 9x13-inch glass dish.

In a large bowl, beat the eggs.

In a food processor, grate the carrots and then the potatoes. Add them to the eggs. Add the oil and salt and pour the whole mixture into the prepared baking dish. Bake for 1 hour.

GRANDMA FRIDA'S POTATO KUGEL

Sandy Glass

"Grandma Frida was born in Chincha, Peru. Her parents, Celinda and Elias Trajtman emigrated from Romania to Peru in the mid-1920s with two children; Frida was the 4th of their 5 children. While Frida Trajtman was babysitting her niece in Panama, she met Bob Brown who was serving in the U.S. Air Force there. They fell in love, married, and moved to New Jersey. Frida made this potato kugel for their three children and later for their grandchildren. I think of Grandma Frida whenever I make this wonderful dish."

Serves 12

6 Yukon gold potatoes, peeled
2 onions
4 eggs, lightly beaten
1/3 cup matzo meal
1 teaspoon salt
1/4 teaspoon pepper
2 tablespoons oil

Preheat the oven to 350°. Grease a 9x13-inch greased baking dish.

Grate the potatoes and onions in a food processor. Add the lightly beaten eggs, matzo meal, salt, pepper, and oil and mix well. Pour the mixture into the prepared baking dish. Bake for 60 minutes, until the top is golden brown.

There were several wonderful noodle kugel recipes submitted, and although all of them couldn't be used, here are a few ideas to enhance your traditional noodle kugel: Irene Arron suggests adding other dried fruits such as apricots, cranberries, or golden raisins to a sweet kugel, and Marcia Shahon uses macaroni instead of the traditional wide egg noodles and combines them with cottage cheese, Romano cheese, American cheese, and Parmesan cheese for a delicious savory kugel.

APRICOT NOODLE PUDDING (KUGEL)

Shirley Rose

Makes 6 to 8 servings

1 8-ounce package wide egg noodles, cooked and drained
4 eggs, well beaten
1 cup sour cream
1 lemon, juiced and rind grated
½ cup butter, melted
½ cup sugar
1 10-ounce jar apricot jam
1 8-ounce carton low fat cottage cheese or plain yogurt (optional)

Preheat the oven to 350°. Butter a 9x9-inch glass baking dish.

Combine the noodles with the eggs, sour cream, lemon juice and lemon rind, melted butter, sugar, jam, salt, and cottage cheese or yogurt and mix well. Turn the mixture into the prepared baking dish and smooth the top. Bake for 1 hour. Watch toward the end of the hour to make sure the top of the kugel doesn't burn. If needed, lower heat or cover loosely with foil to prevent burning.

TIPS & TRICKS:

- I use No Yolks noodles, which come in a 9-ounce package. Cook them for 12 minutes, stirring once or twice.

BLUE RIBBON NOODLE KUGEL

Jan Block

Serves 12 to 16

½ pound medium or extra-wide egg noodles
1 cup unsalted butter, room temperature
1 pound cream cheese, room temperature
1 cup sugar
1 teaspoon vanilla
2 cups sour cream
8 eggs
1 8-ounce can crushed pineapple, drained
1 11-ounce can mandarin oranges, drained and halved

Cook the noodles according to the package directions, drain, and place in a large bowl.

Combine the butter and cream cheese in a food processor and blend until smooth. Add the sugar and blend until well combined. Add the vanilla, sour cream, and eggs and process until smooth. Pour this mixture into the bowl with the cooked noodles.

Stir in the pineapple and oranges by hand. Place the mixture into a buttered 9x13-inch baking dish. It will come to the very top of the dish. Cover and refrigerate overnight for the best results.

Topping:
⅓ cup sugar
4 ounces walnuts, coarsely chopped
1 teaspoon cinnamon
2 tablespoons butter

When ready to bake, preheat the oven to 350°.

Combine the walnuts with the sugar and cinnamon in a small bowl. Sprinkle evenly over the top of the kugel and dot with the 2 tablespoons butter. Bake the kugel for approximately 1 hour or until a knife inserted into the middle comes out clean.

CHICKIE'S KIGGLE*

Marc and David Jacobson

"Her name was Violet Feldman, but everyone always called her Chickie, as she wasn't so fond of the name Violet. She was a remarkable woman, raising four kids on her own on the salary of a Social Security clerical worker. She endured more than her share of tragedies and still remained, to her dying day, a loving, caring, giving, real pistol of a woman. Such a dirty sense of humor, too, for a nice Jewish lady from Northeast Philly.

"Aunt Chickie loved food. Every visit with her revolved around the meals of the day: What were we going to have? Were we going to go out to eat and where?

"I remember her kugel from the time I remember eating. Chickie made it for every holiday and family occasion for her big family, who persist in pronouncing it 'kiggle.'

"I am thrilled not only to have won the Great Kugel Throwdown, but to honor Chickie by bringing her kugel to Seattle, our home for more than five years."

~ Marc Jacobson

Serves 12

8 ounces fine egg noodles
1 cup margarine, softened
1 cup sugar
½ pound cream cheese, softened
2 cups sour cream
2 teaspoons vanilla
8 eggs, beaten
½ to ¾ cup golden raisins
Cinnamon sugar

Preheat the oven to 350°.

Cook the noodles according to package directions, being careful not to overcook. Rinse and drain the noodles.

Cream the margarine and sugar in a large bowl with an electric mixer. Add the cream cheese and mix until smooth. Add the sour cream, vanilla, and eggs, mixing well with each addition.

Mix two-thirds of the custard mixture with the cooked noodles. Add the raisins. Pour the mixture into a greased 9x13-inch glass dish. Gently pour the remaining custard on top. Sprinkle liberally with cinnamon sugar.

Bake for 45 minutes, checking after 40 minutes to be sure it is not getting too brown. It should be lightly browned and evenly spongy to the touch, even in the middle, when it is done. Turn off the oven and leave the dish in the cooling oven for 30 minutes. Remove from the oven and finish cooling or serve warm.

*Chickie's "Kiggle" won the "The Great Kugel Throwdown" held at Hillel at the University of Washington in May 2011. Over 50 people and three judges deemed this kugel the best of 15 kugels prepared by community participants.

MOTHER'S NOODLE KUGEL

Alice Siegal

"As a child in the 1930s, I loved my mother's dairy kugel. I loved the aroma that filled the kitchen, the shiny golden top tinged with brown as it came out of the oven, and the cheesy, custardy taste. Years later as a wife and mother, I realized I had not eaten kugel since I was a child. I had never seen any family recipes, so after much trial and error, I finally achieved what I remembered."

Serves 6 to 8

1 tablespoon butter or margarine
6 ounces wide egg noodles
3 eggs
2 cups low fat cottage cheese
1 cup nonfat yogurt
3 ounces cheddar cheese, grated

Preheat the oven to 350°. Melt the butter and pour into an 8½x11½-inch glass baking dish.

Cook noodles about 10 minutes, rinse with cold water, and drain.

Beat the eggs and then add the cottage cheese, yogurt, and cheddar cheese. Mix well and add the noodles. Pour the kugel mixture into the baking dish.

Bake for about 1 hour, until the top is golden brown.

TIPS & TRICKS:

- The recipe is a sort of basic dairy kugel, which can easily be embellished. Sour cream can be substituted for an equal part of yogurt. For a creamier texture, add 3 ounces of low fat cream cheese. Amounts do not have to be that precise, so it is easy to assemble.

SWEET NOODLE KUGEL

Janet Reis

Serves 12

1 pound wide egg noodles, cooked, drained, and cooled
2½ cups milk
6 eggs, lightly beaten
1 pint cottage cheese (non-fat if preferred)
1½ teaspoons vanilla
1 cup sugar
1 cup golden raisins
2 cups sour cream
¼ cup margarine or butter, melted
1 cup cornflake crumbs, crushed
2 tablespoons sugar
1½ teaspoons cinnamon

In a large bowl, mix the noodles, milk, eggs, cottage cheese, vanilla, sugar, raisins, sour cream, and margarine or butter. Refrigerate overnight.

Preheat the oven to 350°. Butter a 10x15-inch glass baking dish.

Mix the cinnamon and sugar.

Spoon the noodle mixture into the prepared baking dish. Sprinkle the cornflake crumbs and cinnamon-sugar over the kugel. Bake for at least 1 hour, until golden brown and firm to the touch.

MATZO KUGEL

Cynthia Glazer Shifrin

"The way I see it, if cooking isn't a creative expression, it will feel more like a chore: something just needing to get done out of necessity. Cooking and baking were not authentic creative outlets for my mother. I was lucky though to have two grandmothers who were rock stars in the kitchen. I would watch in amazement as they passionately baked and cooked without any written recipes – just instinctively adding some of this and some of that. And voila – everything they prepared was so delish!

"I was also fortunate to have a father who loved to cook and bake. He approached it more as a hobby when time would allow, so it was always a special event whenever he felt inspired. My father's passion for food and his complete enjoyment of being creative in the kitchen were matched and complemented by my mother's passion for eating and her complete enjoyment of everything he prepared.

"Even though my mother was a basic-no-frills-cook, everything she prepared tasted good. What I remember the most was her sweet noodle kugel and matzo brei. Whenever I eat either one of those comfort foods, I'm always reminded of my mother and how loved and nurtured I felt whenever she would prepare them.

"Noodle kugel is a dish I love preparing because of all the tender feelings I associate with it. I always make mine slightly sweet over savory, continuing with family tradition. And I still adore matzo brei topped with maple syrup, just as my mother always served it. I also prepare a sweet matzo kugel that for me is the mother of all comfort foods. It has the same delicate sweetness and rich flavor as my noodle kugel, with the light consistency of a steamed pudding. As soon as I take my very first bite, I'm transported back in memory to being a young girl, even though I have no recollection of anyone in my family preparing sweet kugel with matzo. Perhaps my kugel creativity is being channeled by a distant Eastern European relative – or is buried deep within my cellular memory from a past life – or simply because the foodie in me loves sweet kugel – who knows? Whatever the case, my matzo kugel recipe is one I pass on with all the love in my heart."

Serves 16 to 20

11 sheets matzo, softened in water and drained well
5 eggs
¾ cup plus 1 tablespoon granulated sugar
1 tablespoon vanilla
2 16-ounce containers cottage cheese
1 16-ounce container sour cream
1 cup whole milk
¼ cup butter, melted and cooled
1 large apple, peeled, cored, and finely chopped (optional)
Cinnamon, for sprinkling

Preheat the oven to 350° with the rack placed in the lower third. Grease a 9x13-inch baking dish with butter or a vegetable oil spray.

Break up the matzo into small pieces, place in a colander, and run under very hot water to soften. The consistency should resemble cooked oatmeal. Drain the water by pressing down on the matzo while it's still in the colander.

TIPS & TRICKS:

- The kugel will puff up as it bakes, but will fall when removed from the oven.

In a large bowl, whisk the eggs and sugar, add the vanilla and beat well. Stir in the cottage cheese, sour cream, milk, and cooled butter; add the softened matzo and blend well. Stir in the chopped apples, if using, or any other fruit you'd prefer. Pour the mixture into the prepared baking dish, sprinkle with cinnamon. Bake for 1 hour and 15 minutes. This dish can be prepared a couple days in advance. It also freezes well and can be reheated at 350° for 30 minutes.

MOTHER'S PASSOVER APPLE KUGEL

The Tobin Daughters – Beatrice, Madeline, Goldie, and Lila

"Passover was always special to Mother and Dad and we always enjoyed cooking together. One of the favorites was 'Mother's Apple Kugel.' This recipe can be doubled, as everyone is happy to take home any leftovers.

"When the cooking is finished, the fish is simmering, and the kugel is cooling on a rack, we reward ourselves by opening the first box of matzo and munching on fresh strawberries and cottage cheese."

Serves 8

4 tablespoons butter or margarine
4 eggs, separated
2 cups matzo farfel
4 tart apples, peeled and grated
½ teaspoon salt
½ 6-ounce can orange juice concentrate, frozen
1 teaspoon vanilla (optional)
1 orange, rind grated
2 tablespoons cinnamon-sugar
½ cup walnuts, finely chopped

Preheat the oven to 325°. Melt butter in a 2-quart (8x10-inch) pan.

Beat the egg whites until stiff and set aside. In a large mixing bowl, beat the egg yolks with a whisk until frothy. Rinse the matzo farfel in cold water and drain. Add the matzo farfel, apples, sugar, salt, orange juice concentrate, vanilla, and orange rind and mix well. Fold in the egg whites and pour into the prepared pan. Top with the cinnamon-sugar and walnuts. Bake for 35 minutes, until set.

PASSOVER EGG NOODLES

Morrene Jacobson

"This is the first recipe my husband asked me to get from his mother, Lola Jacobson. You can buy kosher for Passover egg noodles, but they won't taste like these. The recipe is quite labor-intensive. You can easily double or triple the recipe, but be prepared to spend a lot of time on your feet! These noodles are always a part of our Seder meal – yummy, and rich with memories."

Makes 4 servings

4 eggs
4 tablespoons cold water
1/8 teaspoon kosher salt
1 1/2 tablespoons potato starch or matzo cake flour
Canola oil for frying

Beat the eggs, water, and salt until well blended. Using a strainer, sift the potato starch or matzo cake flour into the egg mixture and mix well.

Using a paper towel, wipe the inside of a small nonstick frying pan with oil. Preheat the pan briefly over medium heat. Pour in enough batter to just cover the bottom of the pan. Cook the first side, flip, and cook the second side. Don't overcook – it should be moist and not browned. Cool on a towel and repeat the process with the remainder of the batter, stirring frequently to eliminate lumps.

Stack the circles and cut them in half. Roll each half the short way and make ½-inch slices to cut them into noodles. Add the noodles to your chicken soup, with or without matzo balls

TIPS & TRICKS:

- You can make the noodles ahead and refrigerate them for a day or two. Take them out 1 hour before serving. No need to reheat – just toss them into hot soup.

MATZOH MOMMA'S POTATO LATKES

Pip and Miriam Meyerson

Makes 2 dozen latkes

3 pounds potatoes, peeled (3 to 4 potatoes)
1 onion, minced
3 eggs
3 tablespoons matzo meal or flour
1 teaspoon salt
½ teaspoon pepper
1 cup peanut oil
Applesauce and sour cream, for serving

Grate potatoes (medium grate) into a large bowl. Rinse the potatoes by covering with water and then draining water from mixture, squeezing out as much water as possible.

Add the onions, eggs, matzo meal, salt, and pepper to the potatoes and mix well.

Preheat the peanut oil in large fry pan to medium-high heat (325° to 350°). Ladle out ¼ cup of the latke mixture into the pan and flatten with a spatula. Fry until the edges are golden brown, then flip and cook the other side until brown. Remove and drain on paper towels. Repeat until all the potato mixture is used, adding oil as necessary.

Keep cooked latkes in a warm (250°) oven.

CARROT–SCALLION LATKES

Wendy Lynne

"I love latkes, but I am always looking for a new, healthier version. This one is not only healthy, it is also gluten free since it uses coconut flour instead of regular."

Serves 4

3 cups carrots, shredded
3 scallions (green onions), finely chopped
3 eggs, beaten
½ teaspoon sea salt
½ teaspoon coconut flour, plus more if preferred
Olive oil for frying
Applesauce and sour cream or yogurt, for serving

In a large bowl, combine the carrots, scallions, and eggs. Stir the salt and coconut flour into the carrot mixture.

In a large skillet, heat the olive oil. Scoop heaping tablespoons of batter onto the skillet and fry until brown and crispy. Transfer the latkes to a paper towel-lined plate. Repeat until all the batter is used up.

Serve warm with applesauce and sour cream or yogurt.

BUTTERNUT SQUASH LATKES

Wendy Lynne

"Another healthy latke recipe."

Serves 6

4 cups butternut squash, peeled and grated
1 small onion, peeled and grated
3 eggs, beaten
Grapeseed oil for frying

In a large bowl, mix together the squash, onion, and eggs.

Heat the grapeseed oil in a large skillet. Use your hands to form the batter into 3-inch patties.

Drop the patties into the skillet and fry until they are golden brown and crispy. Remove and drain on paper towel. Repeat until all the batter is used up.

Serve the latkes warm with applesauce, sour cream, or yogurt.

PINK SEPHARDIC RICE

Rachel Almeleh

"I received my first Sephardic cookbook as a wedding gift from my cousin, Mary Halela, in 1970. I began a hobby business in 1993 of taking orders for Sephardic food. At the time, I was still teaching Spanish at Foster High School in Tukwila. Since my mom, Emily Capelouto Almeleh, died when I was just 12, my aunties, Glavina Almeleh, Matty Greenberg, and Rachel Capelouto, taught me the methods of Sephardic cooking not always revealed in cookbooks. My older sister Esther and I attempted our first Sephardic recipe of 'pink rice' for our father, Jacob David Almeleh, shortly after our mother's death. The first attempt was mush and the second, burnt. No matter what, our father ate everything we made. He would say, 'Es pecado,' (a sin, a waste to throw away food). When my cousin, Lucille Almeleh Spring, tasted my food, she said I had 'bendichas manos' (blessed hands). That phrase went on my first business card."

Serves 6

1 cup long grain rice
2 cups water or chicken broth or half of each
1 teaspoon salt
2 tablespoons oil
¼ cup tomato sauce or more if desired

Rinse the rice and drain. Put water or broth, salt, and oil in a saucepan and bring to a boil. Add the rice, return to a boil, and stir. Cover, reduce the heat and simmer for 20 minutes, adding more water if the rice sticks to the pan.

MAUREEN BENOLIEL'S GRANDMOTHER'S RICE

Maureen Benoliel

"My grandmother, who was born on the Isle of Rhodes, was a great cook, and this rice, always a crowd pleaser, is best served with a salad on top. My grandfather was quite strict about following all the rules of holiday services, so they were not always fun, but my grandmother's food made every holiday joyous."

Makes 8 servings

2 cups pearl rice
2/3 cup olive oil
3 cups water
2 teaspoons salt
6 tablespoons tomato sauce
2 15-ounce cans garbanzo beans, drained

Wash and drain the rice three times.

In a large saucepan bring the oil, water, salt, and tomato sauce to a boil. Add the rice and stir. Return to a boil then lower the heat, cover, and simmer for 15 minutes.

Stir in the drained garbanzo beans and continue cooking for another 15 minutes.

TIPS & TRICKS:

- Leftover rice can be refrigerated and is even better reheated the next day.

AUNT ADA'S RICE

Jan Block

"Aunt Ada, who lived to be 102, was a wonderful cook, but preferred to take her favorite recipes to her grave rather than share them! After repeated attempts to get the recipe, my mother finally succeeded one day while on the phone with Aunt Ada. Instead of running to get a piece of paper and taking the risk that Ada would change her mind, my mother tore a page from the phone book and wrote the recipe on that. It is framed and hanging on our kitchen wall today."

Serves 8 to 10

½ cup butter
½ pound fine egg noodles, uncooked
2 cups Minute rice
2 14-ounce cans Campbell's® French onion soup
2 14-ounce cans Campbell's® chicken broth
1 can water
2 tablespoons soy sauce
2 5-ounce cans sliced water chestnuts, drained and chopped

Preheat the oven to 350°.

Melt the butter in a saucepan then brown the noodles in the butter. Add the rice, onion soup, chicken broth, water, soy sauce, and water chestnuts. Stir the mixture and then pour it into a 9x13-inch baking dish.

Bake for 45 minutes.

WILD RICE

Brenda Atkin

"I grew up in Duluth, Minnesota, and my father owned a grocery store. Because of his store, my father was able to get wild rice directly from the Native Americans. This is also why the wild rice had to be washed so many times, as it had not yet been cleaned when my father got it. Today, one probably does not have to wash the wild rice quite as much!

"The Native Americans provided my father and mother with this recipe, and my mother would make it every year for Thanksgiving. I always remember waking up on Thanksgiving morning and going into the kitchen where my mother and I would taste a sample of the wild rice. Now, every time I make this recipe, I stop to take a sample taste and remember back to my childhood when I would share this time with my mother. I also make wild rice every year for Thanksgiving; however, I have expanded on my mother's delicious tradition and also serve it to my family on erev Rosh Hashanah."

Serves 6 to 8

½ pound wild rice
Cold water
2 cups boiling water
1 tablespoon butter
½ green pepper, diced
1 medium onion, diced
1 8-ounce can sliced mushrooms, drained
1 10.5-ounce can cream of mushroom soup

Rinse the wild rice 15 to 20 times in cold water, draining it through a strainer and replacing it with new water each time. Let the rice stand overnight in cold water.

Drain the rice and add the boiling water. Let it sit for 1 hour.

Drain the rice and cover again with boiling water. Let the rice sit for 30 minutes.

Preheat the oven to 350°. Butter an 8x8 glass baking dish.

Melt the butter in a fry pan over medium heat and sauté the green peppers and onions. Add the sliced mushrooms and mushroom soup and stir to combine. Stir in the wild rice. Transfer to the baking dish and bake for 30 minutes.

LENTILS

Esther Sadis

"My mother-in-law, Esther 'Tessie' Sadis, was a wonderful cook. I learned so much from her, especially in the Sephardic delicacies department. When I was first married, she would bake all day, call us over, and we would enjoy every bite of her day's work. When our kids were little, she would get in her car and bring us care packages. As time went on, I decided I really needed to learn how cook to the Sephardic foods she so lovingly prepared. Cooking Sephardic was becoming a dying art and as generous as she was in teaching me, it wasn't ever enough, but after hours and hours of watching her cook, I learned her secrets. When she decided it was too much for her to bake any more, I was able to bring her care packages of all the favorite foods she loved."

Serves 6 to 8

3 to 4 cups water
½ pound lentils
1 small onion, chopped
¼ cup oil
1 8-ounce can tomato sauce
½ teaspoon sugar
2 to 3 bouillon cubes (chicken or vegetarian)
2 stalks celery, chopped
Pinch of pepper

Bring the water to a boil. Pour in the lentils and boil for 2 minutes. Strain, rinse, and set aside.

In the same sauce pan, add the oil and brown the onions. Then add the tomato sauce, sugar, bouillon cubes, celery, and pepper. Sauté for 5 minutes on medium heat then remove from the heat. Add the lentils to the pan and cover with water about 2-inches above the lentils. Bring to a boil, cover, and reduce the heat to medium-low. Cook for 15 minutes and turn off the stove.

TIPS & TRICKS:

- If the mixture becomes too thick, add a little hot water.
- When you reheat lentils, only heat what you plan to eat, not the whole pot. Otherwise, they will turn to mush.

BARLEY PILAF

Bob Rogers

2 servings

2 tablespoons margarine
2 tablespoons pine nuts
3 green onions, chopped (including most of the greens)
½ cup barley
1 tablespoon parsley, chopped
Salt and pepper, to taste
1¾ cups chicken broth, heated

Preheat the oven to 350°.

Lightly brown pine nuts in margarine. Remove and reserve. In the same pan, sauté the barley and green onions until the barley is lightly toasted. Remove from heat. Add the nuts, parsley, salt, and pepper and stir. Pour the hot broth over the barley and stir.

Transfer the mixture to a covered 2-quart casserole and bake for about 1 to 1¼ hours. The barley should be moist but not runny.

GRANDMA'S AVECAS

Maggie Halela Mosholder and Rebecca Peterson

"Our Grandma Benveniste was an amazing woman who came to the United States from Istanbul when she was 17 years old. She was a self-taught woman who knew a variety of languages and was an excellent cook. My cousins and I laugh about the many times we would try to ask her to teach us recipes by using the traditional 'cup' and 'teaspoon' methods. She would get annoyed and say 'use three eggs' or 'this much' (holding up a jelly jar). Obviously she had all the recipes in her head, but we were able to decipher a few that we are happy to prepare today, and remember her and the never-ending amount of love she had for us all."

Serves 6

1 cup dried white beans (Great Northern)
1 medium onion, diced
3 tablespoons oil
½ small can tomato sauce

Place the white beans in a large pot and cover with water. Boil over medium heat, adding water as the beans expand and water lowers. Cook for at least 1 hour.

Sauté the onion in the oil over low heat. Once the onions have softened, add the tomato sauce and simmer.

Rinse the beans and add them to the sauce. Cover the beans with water and cook for 2 to 3 hours on low heat, until the beans are tender. The beans can also be baked in a 325° oven for the same amount of time.

TIPS & TRICKS:

- A shortcut for these beans would be to use two 15-ounce cans of cannellini beans (drained), mix them with the onion, oil, and tomato sauce and bake for 1 hour, until they are tender.

POTATOES ROMANOFF

Laura Oseran Miller

"My mother, *Sylvia Oseran, made Potatoes Romanoff every Rosh Hashanah dinner and Passover Seder for over 30 years. With just a hint of heat, it is a creamy and cheesy side dish that goes particularly well with salmon.*"

Serves 16

3 20-ounce packages Simply Potatoes Shredded Hashed Browns
4 cups sour cream
3 bunches green onions, sliced
4 cups cheddar cheese, shredded and divided
3 teaspoons garlic powder
2 to 3 teaspoons Tabasco sauce (depending on how hot you like it)
1 teaspoon salt
Pepper
Paprika

Preheat the oven to 350°. Butter a 10x15-inch glass dish.

In a large bowl, combine the potatoes, sour cream, green onions, 3 cups of the cheddar cheese, garlic powder, Tabasco sauce, and salt. Season to taste with pepper. Pour the mixture into the baking dish and top with the remaining cup of cheddar cheese. Sprinkle with paprika.

Bake for 40 to 45 minutes, until nicely browned on the top.

TIPS & TRICKS:

- You can find the Simply Potatoes Shredded Hash Browns in the refrigerated section of your grocery store.

FOUR CHEESE RIGATONI

Anne Masin

"Some people might call this dish 'mac and cheese,' but we call it delicious. Food doesn't get any more comforting than this."

Serves 10 to 12

1 pound rigatoni
1 pound sharp cheddar cheese, grated
1 pound mozzarella cheese, grated
3¾ cups 2% milk
7 tablespoons butter
½ cup flour
½ cup Parmesan cheese, grated
¼ cup Romano cheese, grated
1 teaspoon Tabasco sauce
¼ teaspoon white pepper, heaping
¾ teaspoon chili powder

Cook the rigatoni for 4 to 6 minutes. Drain and set aside.

Combine the cheddar and mozzarella cheeses. Set aside.

For the béchamel sauce, heat 3 cups of the milk until just about boiling in the microwave or in a small saucepan on the stove.

In a large saucepan, melt the butter over medium heat. After the foam subsides, remove the pan from the heat and add the flour. Mix well and reduce heat to low. Cook the butter and flour mixture for 2 to 3 minutes, being careful not to brown. Add the hot milk slowly and stir until the mixture has thickened and is smooth, 3 minutes or so. Add the Parmesan and Romano cheeses and whisk again. Then blend in the Tabasco sauce and white pepper.

Fold the rigatoni into the béchamel.

Preheat the oven to 375°.

TIPS & TRICKS:

- This can be made the day before, covered with plastic wrap, and stored in the refrigerator. Bring it to room temperature before baking.
- It can even be frozen. Just add 20 minutes to baking time.
- Make sure it is piping hot by testing the noodles in the middle of the casserole.

To assemble, spoon half of the rigatoni mixture into a 9x13-inch ovenproof dish. Top with half of the cheese mixture. Spoon the remaining rigatoni and then the rest of the cheese mixture. Sprinkle chili powder over the top.

When ready to bake, pour the remaining ¾ cup of milk over the casserole. Set the macaroni and cheese into the oven and bake for 1 hour. Watch the top so it doesn't burn, but it should be dark golden brown and crispy.

FARFALLE WITH KALE, CURRANTS, AND PINENUTS

Kathy Fishman

"This vegetarian dish is very popular with my family and as hearty as it is healthy."

Serves 6

1 pound farfalle pasta
2 tablespoons kosher salt
¾ cup dried currants
2 bunches kale, well-washed
½ cup oil
¾ cup pine nuts
6 cloves garlic, sliced
2 teaspoons kosher salt
1 teaspoon pepper

Boil the pasta in salted water for about 7 minutes. Drain, reserving 1 cup of the liquid, and allow the pasta to cool.

Pour the reserved pasta water over the currants, allowing them to soften while you prepare the other ingredients.

Cut the kale into chiffonade by rolling the leaves into cigar-like bundles and cutting across into ¼-inch ribbons.

Put the oil in a large sauté pan over medium heat and cook pine nuts for about 2 minutes, until light brown. Lightly brown the garlic and then add the kale and sauté for 2 minutes.

Drain the currants and add to the kale, then toss with the pasta. Season with the salt and pepper.

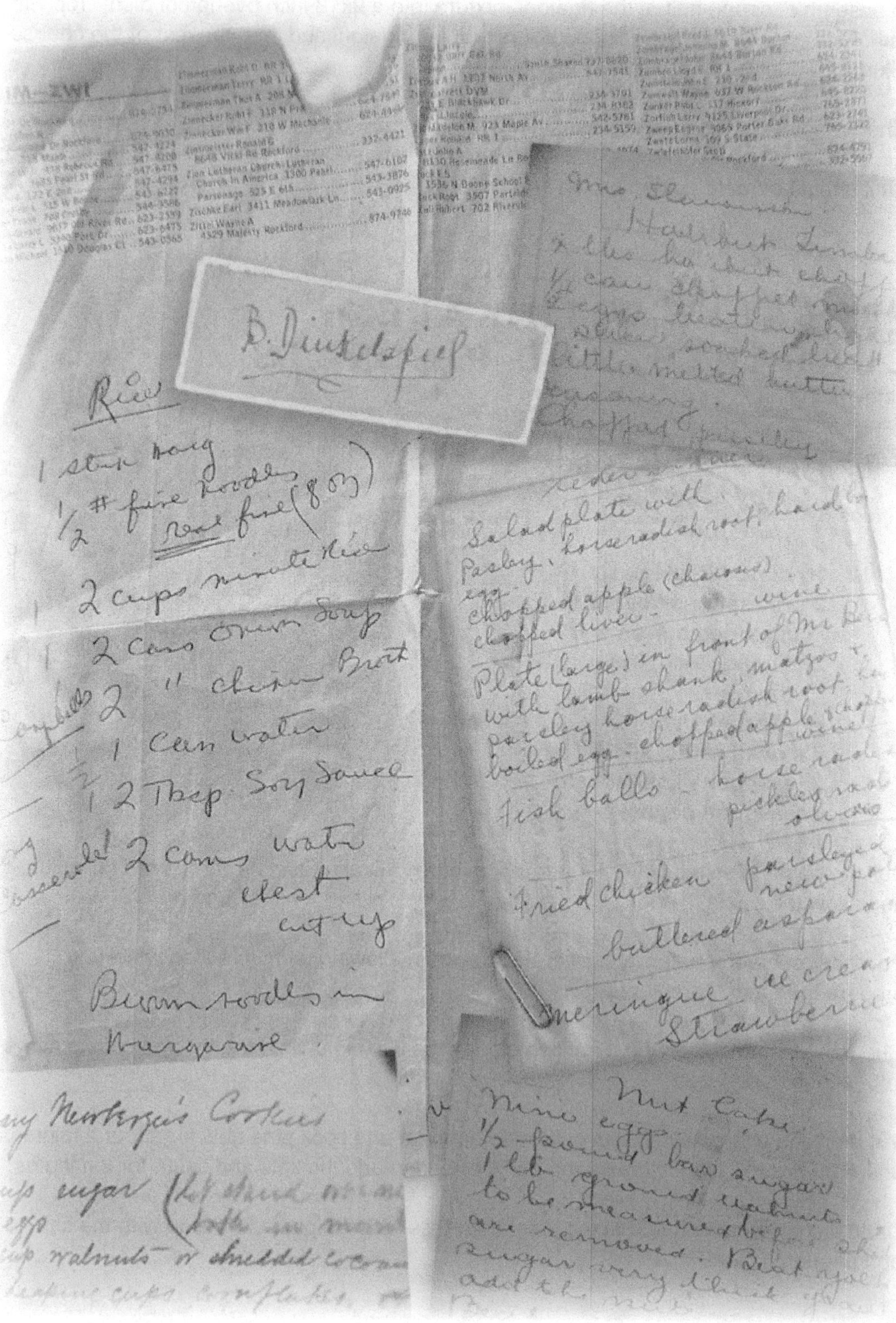

B. Dinkelspiel
Rice
1 stick marg
1/2 # fine noodles
real fine (8 oz)
2 cups minute Rice
2 Cans Onion Soup
2 " chicken Broth
1 Can water
2 Tbsp Soy Sauce
2 cans water
Brown noodles in Margarine
Salad plate with
Parsley, horseradish root, hard boiled egg
chopped apple (charoses)
chopped liver
wine
Plate (large) in front of Mr B
with lamb shank, matzos
parsley horseradish root
boiled egg. chopped apple
Fish balls
horseradish
pickles
olives
Fried chicken
parsleyed new potatoes
buttered asparagus
meringue
ice cream
Strawberries
Nut Cake
Nine eggs
1/2 pound bar sugar
1 lb ground walnuts
to be measured before shells are removed.

Meatballs to Meghina

Meat has long been the centerpiece of traditional Jewish meals. While modern-day foodies have taken liberties to reinvent the classics with vegetarian substitutions, exotic marinades, and cooking methods, or local, sustainable ingredients (or all of the above), chicken, beef, and lamb are typically the central foci around which the other dishes are merely supporting roles.

Gastronomic creativity aside, the preparation of meat and the parts of the animal used have changed over the course of American Jewish history. Some old-time delicacies, such as calf liver and beef tongue, seem to have gone the way of the wall-mounted dial telephone; others ebb and flow in and out of vogue with modern adaptations; others yet are as old and virtually unchanged as the hills.

Brisket and its first cousins pastrami and corned beef are mainstays in Jewish homes and delis, particularly of the Ashkenazi variety. Norma Rosenthal meditates on her father's corned beef recipe, which appeared at every family event and whose preparation was so involved that cooking became a ritual itself. Leslie Huppin upgrades the traditional brisket with succulent flavors that invoke a Memphis barbeque – though Jews live everywhere, there's hardly such a thing as Memphis Jewish cooking. But can't we assume that our descendants will one day reminisce about such localized American-Jewish recipes as these?

Speaking of innovation, Jordan Lott updates the common chicken – a "Jewish meat" if there ever was one – with his Beer Can Chicken, which calls for coriander and sesame seeds among a host of other vibrant flavors and, yes, beer. Another young "foodie" is also among the most adventurous: Brooke Benaroya Dickson takes the traditional chicken to new heights with fennel, figs, and a North African spice blend. Betsy Schneier's mother's Chicken Teriyaki, inspired by a stream of foreign exchange students from Asia, is a foodie recipe of another generation, and Craig Sternberg's "Shabbat cooking for men" experience subtly reminds us that the times are constantly changing.

While we might pride ourselves on these advances, the stories here remind us of the comforts we possess. Hilda Preuss' One Pot Meal is overshadowed by her perilous escape from Europe. Henriett Arditti Hasson is remembered for her *meghina* and for being a multilingual Tunisian immigrant with a small stature and an infectious laugh. Edith Morgan passed down her Hungarian recipes and expert tips without ever writing anything out. May we all be so lucky to cook as well and live as long, with or without the paprika and *potchka*.

MEATBALLS TO MEGHINA

HILLIARD GOLDEN'S CORNED BEEF

Norma Rosenthal

"This is my father's family's favorite recipe for corned beef. I can't remember any celebration or life cycle event that didn't include this dish...from my childhood growing up in Portland, Oregon, to my grown daughters' bat mitzvahs and wedding celebrations. Because the entire process of corning the beef took so long, it was a ritual itself. Once it was sliced and served, we would savor every bite. Of course, it is best when accompanied by what my Dad calls 'real' Jewish rye bread (which excludes anything from the grocery store shelf and can only be found at a 'real' Jewish deli) and the best yellow mustard you can find. Just talking about it makes my mouth water and brings back so many memories."

Serves 12 to 15

5 pounds of beef brisket, extra lean
½ cup kosher salt
3 cloves garlic, slivered
3 tablespoons whole mixed pickling spices
1 teaspoon sugar
½ teaspoon saltpeter
2 cups water

Make small slits in the brisket (about 3 inches apart) and insert slivers of garlic. Mix the pickling spices, sugar, saltpeter, and water in a crock and add the meat. Cover. Store in the refrigerator and soak for 10 days, turning the meat twice during the process. Make sure the meat is submerged in the liquid. (You can place a small plate face down over the meat with a clean brick or some other heavy object on top.)

Soak the pickled meat in cold water for one hour. Remove from cold water and place in a pan with a lid large enough to hold the 5-pound piece of corned beef. Cover the meat with fresh water and simmer for 3 hours or until a fork stuck into the middle of the meat comes out easily. Cool and sprinkle with paprika. Wrap in plastic wrap and then foil to store in the refrigerator. Slice very thin to serve.

HELENE'S SWEET AND SOUR CORNED BEEF

Cindy Stratiner, Alan Waldbaum, and Ron Waldbaum

"When we were young, we had many a fun Sunday night dinner at our Grandma Helene's home. This corned beef recipe was just one of our family's favorites that she often made. Grandma lived in a warm, brick home on Capitol Hill, not far from where she had grown up as the oldest of nine children of the large Rogers brood. Being part of a large family probably contributed to her always entertaining a group for dinner, not only for holidays, but on many Sunday nights. She would usually include friends, siblings, nieces, nephews, cousins, or someone who was new to town. Her three boys and their families were always included. Then later when she married her second husband, Mac Sprincin, it was 'the more the merrier,' as Grandma always included her stepsons and their families. We loved having all the cousins to hang and play with as we ran around the house or watched TV on her bed. Grandma Helene always kept a box of See's Candy on her nightstand for dessert!"

Serves 10

6 to 8 pound piece center cut corned beef
12 ounces water or 1 12-ounce can Coca-Cola®

Preheat the oven to 325°.

Place the corned beef in a large ovenproof container with a lid. Cover the meat with the water or Coca-Cola®. Bake the corned beef, no matter the size, for 3 hours. The last ½ hour of cooking, add the sauce.

Sauce:
3 tablespoons margarine or oil
3 tablespoons white vinegar
3 tablespoons water
⅓ cup ketchup
⅓ cup brown sugar
1 tablespoon yellow mustard

In a small sauce pan, melt the margarine or oil. Add the white vinegar, water, ketchup, brown sugar, and yellow mustard. Whisk to blend all of the ingredients together. Pour sauce over the corned beef.

Cook the corned beef for another ½ hour, slice, and serve hot.

BEEF BRISKET

Leslie Huppin

"We've tried many brisket recipes, but I have to say this is my favorite. It is so flavorful, tasting almost like beef you would eat at a Memphis barbecue."

Serves 8 to 10

8 pounds beef brisket
3 large yellow onions, chopped
1 pound carrots, peeled and sliced into ¾-inch chunks
3 heads garlic, peeled and separated
2 2-ounce packages dry onion soup mix
2 12-ounce bottles Heinz® chili sauce
2 16.9-ounce bottles Coca-Cola®

Preheat the oven to 350°.

Spray the inside of a large roasting pan with non-stick spray. Place the brisket in the pan on top of the stove and braise it on both sides until golden brown.

Remove the pan from the stove and place the onions, carrots, and garlic all around the meat. Spread the onion soup mix over the meat and rub it in. Pour the chili sauce over the meat and then pour the Coca-Cola® around the meat.

Cover the pan very tightly with foil and bake at 350° for 5 hours. Let the meat cool completely and then slice. Return the meat to the pan and continue baking at 350° for 1 hour, covered.

TIPS & TRICKS:

- Once cooked and cooled, the brisket can be frozen for later use (but do not slice before storing).
- Check the brisket to be sure there is enough sauce. You may need to add 1 cup of water when returning the brisket to the pan for the last

BRISKET WITH ORANGE JUICE AND DATES

Patty Friedman

Serves 8

5 pounds beef brisket
Salt and pepper
4 teaspoons sugar
3 tablespoons olive oil, plus more for searing
1 pound onions, thinly sliced
1/3 cup red wine vinegar
1/2 teaspoon allspice
2 cups low sodium chicken broth (or 1 cup chicken broth and 1 cup beer)
1 cup orange juice, freshly squeezed (preferable)
1/2 cup tomato sauce
2 cups pitted dates
1 large handful parsley, finely chopped

Preheat the oven to 350°.

Sprinkle the brisket on all sides with salt, pepper, and sugar. In a Dutch oven, heat olive oil over medium heat and sear the meat until browned on all sides. Transfer to a plate. Add the 3 tablespoons of olive oil and onions to the same pan and sauté until dark brown (not burnt), 10 to 15 minutes. Add vinegar and allspice and boil until onion mixture is reduced to a glaze. Add the broth (or broth and beer), orange juice, and tomato sauce and bring to a boil. Return brisket to the pot with the mixture. Scatter the dates around and sprinkle with parsley.

Cover the Dutch oven and place it in the oven for 2½ hours or until tender. If preparing in advance, slice the brisket and place it back in the Dutch oven with the sauce until ready to reheat and serve.

BEEF RIBS SUPREME

Kenny Alhadeff

"These were my favorite ribs, ever. When I knew we were having them, I would skip lunch at school. The moment I came through the front door and smelled them, I got excited. To this day I can smell and taste them in my mind and heart, and it opens a flood gate of joyous memories of my mother, Joan Alhadeff. Food is life, but it often represents love."

Serves 6

½ cup soy sauce
2 cloves garlic
4 tablespoons bourbon whiskey
1 tablespoon olive oil
2 tablespoons honey
2 teaspoons Worcestershire Sauce
2 teaspoons vinegar
2 teaspoons steak Sauce
2 teaspoons ketchup
6 to 8 pounds beef ribs

Mix the soy sauce, garlic, whiskey, olive oil, honey, Worcestershire sauce, vinegar, steak sauce, and ketchup together in a medium bowl. Pour the mixture over the ribs and marinate for several hours.

When ready to cook, preheat the oven to 350°. Cover and bake for 3 hours, basting and turning every 45 minutes.

ENGLISH SHORT RIBS

Roly Alhadeff

Serves 6 to 8

3 pounds meaty short ribs, in three-inch pieces
½ teaspoon salt
½ teaspoon pepper
½ teaspoon garlic powder
1 tablespoon dried minced onion

Sauce:
3 tablespoons soy sauce
1 clove garlic, minced
½ teaspoon ground ginger
⅓ cup white vinegar
⅓ cup brown sugar
¾ cup pineapple juice
3 8-ounce cans tomato sauce

Sprinkle the ribs with the salt, pepper, garlic powder, and minced onion. Allow the ribs to sit in a covered Dutch oven at room temperature for 2 hours.

When ready to cook, preheat the oven to 400°. Uncover the Dutch oven, place it inside the oven, and roast the short ribs for 1 hour.

Prepare the sauce while the meat cooks. Mix the soy sauce, garlic, ginger, vinegar, brown sugar, pineapple juice, and tomato sauce in a sauce pan and simmer for 30 minutes.

Pour ½ of the sauce over the ribs, recover the Dutch oven, reduce temperature to 300°, and bake for approximately 3 hours, basting occasionally, until the meat is very tender.

Pass the remaining sauce with the prepared ribs.

BUBIE'S MEATBALLS

Molly Cone

"One of the many cooking tips I received from my mother-in-law, this recipe is my most valued. She called it a 'meal in one dish.' These meatballs are simple to make, light in texture, and a guaranteed family favorite."

Makes 12 large or 24 small meatballs

1 large potato, peeled and cut into chunks
1 large onion, peeled and cut into chunks
2 garlic cloves, peeled
2 pounds ground beef, lean
1 egg
1 teaspoon kosher salt
1 teaspoon black pepper
1/4 to 1/3 cup matzo meal (or fine dry bread crumbs)
1/2 to 1 cup water

In a food processor, chop the potato, onion, and garlic (not too fine). Transfer mixture to a large bowl. Add the ground beef, egg, salt, and pepper. Mix together by hand or with a large fork. Add matzo meal (or bread crumbs) and mix again. Add water as necessary to form a light, but workable, mixture.

Roll mixture to the desired size and sauté in olive oil, shaking the pan often. Turn the meatballs from side to side until well-browned and move to a serving dish.

TIPS & TRICKS:

- The meatballs can also be served with fresh mushrooms mixed with pan drippings.
- You can make a mushroom sauce by sautéing mushrooms in the pan and adding 1 cup of cold chicken broth that has been whisked with a tablespoon of flour. Simmer, stirring often, until well-blended and lightly thickened.
- Try adding a small can of mushroom steak sauce to the pan drippings.

SWEET 'N SOUR SAUCE FOR MEATBALLS

Roly Alhadeff

"This wonderful recipe is from my mother, Dori Alhadeff's, private collection of favorite recipes."

Makes 6 cups

1/3 cup boysenberry jelly
1 14-ounce can stewed tomatoes
1 28-ounce can whole tomatoes
1 4-ounce can tomato paste
1 onion, finely chopped
2 tablespoons lemon juice
4 tablespoons brown sugar
1 14-ounce bottle ketchup

Combine the boysenberry jelly, stewed tomatoes, whole tomatoes, tomato paste, onion, lemon juice, brown sugar, and ketchup and simmer the mixture for 30 minutes.

Add your favorite prepared meatballs to the sauce and simmer until the meatballs are heated throughout.

TIPS & TRICKS:

- You can use beef or turkey meatballs.

MEGHINA (MEAT PIE)

Doreen Alhadeff

"Passover would not be Passover without this meghina that my grandmother and mother made every year."

Serves 12 to 16

2 pounds ground beef (1 pound regular and 1 pound lean)
2 medium onions, chopped
1 tablespoon salt
2 teaspoons pepper
¼ cup fresh parsley, chopped
2 cups water
12 eggs
Pinch of salt
6 to 9 sheets matzo, plus more as needed

Brown the ground beef in a wide sauté pan. When most of the red is gone, add the salt, pepper, and onion and cook 15 more minutes. Add the 2 cups of water and cook over medium-low heat for 2 hours, breaking up the clumps of meat during cooking. When finished, the meat should be soft and the water should be absorbed. Spoon off as much of the fat as possible and allow meat to cool.

Soak 3 matzos at a time in warm water for 3 minutes. Squeeze out the liquid. In a shallow bowl, beat 3 eggs and add a pinch of salt. Combine the soaked and squeezed matzo with the eggs, mixing very well. (The mixture should be sufficiently stiff to "line" the sides and bottom of the pan. Repeat the process if necessary, as additional matzo may be needed.)

Spray a 9x13-inch glass dish and use ½ the egg and matzo mixture to line the bottom and sides of the dish, forming a crust.

Check the meat mixture and see if additional grease or liquid can be removed. Mix again and break up any clumps of meat. Add the fresh parsley and at least 5 beaten eggs, adding more eggs until the meat and eggs are mixed thoroughly. Pour the egg and meat mixture into the matzo crust and then top with any remaining mixture, making more if necessary.

Bake at 350° for 45 minutes until golden and bubbling. Cut into squares and serve hot or warm.

TIPS & TRICKS:

- Squeeze some lemon juice over the top.

MEGHINA

Eileen Kulman

"My Grandma, Henriett Arditti Hasson, was born in 1910 in Tunis, Tunisia. She was raised in Paris, France, and came to the United States at 18 years of age. She used her sister's passport to enter the country because her sister wanted to stay in Paris to get married. She spoke six languages, and they wanted her to stay on Ellis Island to translate for them, but she settled in San Francisco where her uncle was already living. She later moved to Seattle to be closer to her family. She was a wonderful seamstress, awesome cook and baker, and mother of two. She taught herself English through the dictionary, but continued to have a thick French accent, which we all loved. She stood all of 4' 11", but she was a pistol and had this wonderfully contagious laugh. The most important thing in her life was her family. She loved to be surrounded by family and always had us all over for big family dinners. She died when she was 90, but she lives on in all of us. The following Meghina recipe was one of her favorites."

Serves 12

2 pounds ground beef
2 large onions, chopped
5 cloves garlic, minced
2 tablespoons olive oil
½ cup water
Salt and pepper to taste
4 eggs, beaten

Preheat the oven to 375°.

Combine the beef, onions, garlic, oil, and water in a large skillet. Cover and simmer slowly over low heat, stirring frequently for approximately 1 hour. Season with salt and pepper. Remove from the heat and cool.

Add the eggs to the cooled meat mixture and pour into a greased 9x13-inch pan. Bake for 30 minutes until nicely browned. Remove from the oven and cool for 5 minutes before cutting into pieces.

TIPS & TRICKS:

- This recipe may be used as an appetizer by cutting the meghina into smaller pieces.

NANCY AND GERTRUDE'S SOUTHERN STYLE MEATLOAF

Michele Rosen

"While this recipe is an import from South Carolina, it is a good one for those bone-chilling Seattle nights."

Serves 8

1 pound ground beef
1 pound ground veal
1 onion, finely chopped
3 to 4 cloves garlic, finely chopped
2 eggs, beaten
½ to ¾ cup bread crumbs
1 teaspoon salt
1 10½-ounce can tomato soup or good quality tomato sauce

Preheat the oven to 350°.

Combine the beef, veal, onion, garlic, eggs, bread crumbs, and salt in a large mixing bowl and mix well. Mound the mixture into a 9x5-inch loaf pan. Pour and spread the tomato soup or tomato sauce over the meat mixture and bake for 1 hour.

STUFFED ONIONS (SEVOYAS REYNADAS)

Katherine Scharhon

Serves 6 to 8

4 to 6 medium onions, cut in half laterally (not through the roots)
1 pound ground hamburger meat
Pinch of salt
½ teaspoon pepper
1 egg
2 slices of bread, crumbled into breadcrumbs
½ cup parsley, finely chopped
1 cup onion, finely chopped
1 15-ounce can tomato sauce
Matzo meal, for dipping (or flour)
1 egg, beaten
Vegetable oil, for frying

Preheat the oven to 350°.

Cut the onions in half and remove the first 4 interior onion "shells" from the middle of each cut side. Chop the shells and set aside.

Mix the hamburger, salt, pepper, egg, breadcrumbs, parsley, and 1 cup of the onion. Stuff the half onions with the meat mixture. Dip the stuffed side into matzo meal, then into the beaten egg, and fry in the heated vegetable oil until just browned.

Layer the bottom of an ovenproof sauté pan with the remaining chopped onion and ½ cup tomato sauce.

Place the stuffed onions meat-side up on the tomato sauce and pour the remaining tomato sauce over them. Add enough water to cover the meat. Cover sauté pan with the lid and either bake in the oven at 350° for 45 minutes or cook on the stove top until tender.

EDITH MORGAN'S STUFFED PEPPERS

Linda Morgan

"My mother-in-law, Edith Morgan, never really had a formal recipe for her wonderful stuffed peppers. She claims it was common to not have written recipes in Hungary, where she grew up.

"Stuffed peppers are merely a sample of the Eastern European cuisine Edith often created for the family. There was veal loaf, chicken paprikash, goulash of every variety, Wiener schnitzel, stuffed cabbage, plum cake, and sponge cake. Nearly every recipe, with the exception of the cakes, of course, shared a common ingredient: paprika. Most also included green peppers. It wasn't until our family journeyed to Budapest that we understood these two items, paprika and green pepper, to be Hungarian staples. I learned to make this delectable dish in the 70s, early in my marriage. But, needing an update, I recently asked Edith for a few refresher tips.

"'Don't put too much rice,' said Edith, now 90 years old. 'Leave a little room because the rice puffs up when it cooks. When you cut the top of the peppers off, put them in the pot; it adds good flavor. And remember, you can prepare this all ahead of time, because it's a potchka *to make.'"*

Serves 4 to 6

2 pounds ground beef
4 to 6 large green peppers
1 onion, chopped
½ cup uncooked rice
1 egg
Salt and pepper to taste
2 15-ounce cans tomato sauce
1 tablespoon sugar

Clean out the green peppers, cutting just the tops off, and placing them in a pot large enough to hold all the peppers. Mix the ground beef with the rice, egg, chopped onion, salt, and pepper (or other seasoning of your choice) to taste. Fill each pepper with the beef mixture. Put in a large pot and cover the peppers with tomato sauce. Sprinkle with sugar. Cover, bring to a boil, then cook on simmer until the meat is cooked through, about 50 minutes.

PRAKAS

Edie Bean

"I have created my prakas *based on recipes I've seen in cookbooks, combined with the flavors I remember from my mother's praka recipe. She used citric acid in her recipe, and I use lemon juice. I prefer a sweeter taste than she preferred, and I always put some of the meat mixture inside the two halves of one green pepper and place those in with the prakas while cooking. The green pepper adds a certain flavor I love."*

Makes 25 to 30 prakas

2 large heads of cabbage
2 pounds ground beef
1 egg, beaten
1 small onion, grated
⅔ cup uncooked rice
2 teaspoons salt
Pepper to taste

Remove the leaves from the heads of cabbage and steam over boiling water. Soak the leaves until pliable and then drain.

Combine the meat, onion, rice, salt, egg, and pepper. Place ¼ to ⅓ cup of the meat mixture in each cabbage leaf. Tuck in the sides as you roll up each praka and secure with a toothpick.

Sauce:
1 28-ounce can tomatoes
2½ cups water
1 large onion, chopped
1 teaspoon salt
1 8-ounce can tomato sauce
Lemon juice, to taste
Brown sugar, to taste

In a Dutch oven, combine the tomatoes, water, onion, salt, and tomato sauce. Add the lemon juice and brown sugar to taste. Bring to a boil and simmer for 30 minutes.

Place the cabbage rolls in the sauce in the Dutch oven, cover, and simmer gently for at least 3 hours – the longer the better.

TIPS & TRICKS:

- If preferred, the prakas can be placed in the oven at 350° and baked for 3 hours.

"My recipe for prakas (or proccas) came from my Russian grandmother, Rose Barde Simon, born in Odessa in 1880. She married my grandfather, Ben Simon, and they lived in Portland, Oregon, from 1898, until Ben's death in 1943. Then Rose moved to Los Angeles, California, to be close to her daughters. Grandma Rose taught me and my mother, Daisy Simon Rafish, how to make prakas. My mother married Sam Rafish in Portland in 1930, and they lived in Butte, Montana, until they died. The recipe was printed in 1976 in Butte's Heritage Cookbook, by the Butte-Silver Bow County Bicentennial Commission. It contains recipes from members of at least 14 different cultures living in Butte, Montana."

~ Frankie Bookey

YAPRACKS WITH MEAT AND BEANS

Esther Maimon

"My mother, Sema Calvo, was an incredible cook and baker. When you sat down at her table (for a holiday or otherwise), you knew you were in for a treat. Her meals were always delicious, usually Sephardic in nature, and prepared with love. Each meal nearly always ended with a cup of coffee and a plate of her wonderful biscochos. The recipe that I have submitted is one of my favorite Sephardic dishes that she would often prepare – yapracks with meat and beans."

1 jar grape leaves
1 tablespoon olive oil

Drain the grape leaves and separate the torn and tough leaves from the good ones. Set them aside. (Those leaves will be used to line the bottom of the pan to prevent the rolled leaves from sticking.) Remove the tough stems from the remaining leaves.

Filling:
1 small to medium onion
Olive oil
1 egg
¼ cup parsley, chopped
3 tablespoons uncooked rice (on Passover substitute matzo meal)
1 pound ground beef, lean
Salt and pepper
1 15-ounce can garbanzo beans, drained

Sauté the onion in a small amount of olive oil and cool. Add the egg, parsley, uncooked rice, and ground beef. Season with salt and pepper.

Fill each grape leaf with 1 tablespoon of the meat mixture and roll with ends tucked in (not too tightly as rice will expand).

Grease the bottom of the dish. Place some of the torn and tough leaves in the bottom of the dish and add a tablespoon of oil. Place yapracks on top of the leaves, starting with the outer edge of the pan and working inwards. Sprinkle garbanzo beans on top of the yapracks. Add a second and third layer, if necessary, with garbanzo beans between the layers.

Sauce:
1 tablespoon oil
1 teaspoon sugar
1 to 1½ lemons, juiced
1 8-ounce can tomato sauce
⅛ to ¼ cup water
½ teaspoon salt

Mix the oil, sugar, lemon juice, tomato sauce, water, and salt in a small bowl and pour the sauce over the yapracks. Cover the yapracks with the remaining leaves. Place a dish face-side down on top of the leaves and cover the pan with a lid.

Cook the yapracks on top of the stove on low heat first, then medium heat. Simmer, until tender, approximately 30 to 45 minutes.

If the sauce is too runny, uncover the pot until the excess liquid evaporates.

HILDA'S ONE POT MEAL (KOHL)

Jane Preuss

"My mother-in-law was strong and opinionated. She did everything 200%. Sometimes, we saw eye-to-eye, and sometimes we did not, but we could always count on good times in the kitchen. Since day one, Hilda's recipes have been my family's favorites; my daughter always requested this particular recipe for her birthday. I might add that it was a lot of work because in the early days, we used a hand grinder. Today's modern conveniences make this a fast and delicious meal.

"Hilda's tenacity and determination saved her life as well as the lives of her son and husband. In 1938, right before Hitler took over Austria, Hilda's ex-husband (they had recently been divorced) was arrested by the Nazis. Hilda immediately set off to rescue him, leaving her 1½-year old son, Peter, with her mother. Hilda first traveled to Belgium and unsuccessfully searched for him through two deportation centers. Eventually, she found and liberated him from Dachau concentration camp in Germany. Since Vienna was so dangerous, they lived in Belgium for two years until her husband was again arrested and taken to a concentration camp. Again, Hilda secured his release. She and Peter then fled to Paris and, finally, in 1941, with her brother, they traveled by train to a small town near the Spanish border. A guide led them on a 3-day trek over the Pyrenees Mountains. Hilda's brother carried 2½-year old Peter the entire way. As they crossed the border into Spain, the police arrested the adults and held them in prison as illegal refugees; nuns took Peter to a Catholic hospice for orphans. They were all released after about 5 months and then made their way to Barcelona.

"Since Hilda had no relatives in America to sponsor her, she needed an affidavit from someone in the United States attesting to a source of support. Upon her release from prison, she went to the U.S. Embassy in Barcelona. While there, she looked through the telephone books of major U.S. cities. In them, she found 10 people with her maiden name and 10 with her married name. Hilda wrote a letter to each of them explaining she needed a sponsor. She received one offer, which was all she needed. She and Peter were off to New York City in 1944.

"In 1949, Hilda answered a personals ad in the German language newspaper from a man in Portland, Oregon, who was originally from Berlin and had spent the war years in Shanghai with his son Rolf who was 2 years older than Peter. After a short correspondence, Hilda and Peter boarded the train to Portland. Soon thereafter, she and Adi Preuss, the great love of her life, married. They enjoyed having parties at their new home; Hilda cooked and Adi played the piano. Hilda's cooking was legendary; friends of my husband, Rolf, from his University of Washington days, still reminisce about driving to Portland specifically for one of Hilda's great meals."

Serves 4 to 6

8 cups water
1 head curly cabbage (Savoy), cut into 8 to 10 chunks with the hard center portion removed
1 very large or 2 smaller potatoes, peeled and cut into quarters
1 or 2 tablespoons caraway rye seeds
2 cloves garlic, minced
¼ cup olive oil
2 to 3 tablespoons flour
1 or 2 large sausage(s), fully cooked and sliced into 1-inch pieces (optional)

Bring water to a boil in a large pot. Add the cabbage, potatoes, and caraway seeds and cook for 5 minutes. Pour out all but 1 inch of the water. Cook the potatoes until done, about 30 minutes. Drain all the liquid from the pot, leaving the cooked cabbage and potatoes.

Place the cabbage and potatoes in a food processor fitted with the metal blade and pulse the vegetables until still chunky, but not soupy.

Make a roux by heating the oil over a low heat, adding the minced garlic and flour until mixture is thickened and has turned light yellow. If the mixture is too thin, add additional flour. Add the roux to the cabbage and potato mixture and season with salt and pepper. Add the sausage, if desired, and serve with dense peasant bread.

MOROCCAN LAMB BURGERS

Kathy Fishman

"This recipe is new to me, but it will become a regular in my repertoire of favorite recipes. The patties can be made much smaller and served as an appetizer when put on a dollar roll or even inside a wedge of pita with a dollop of sauce."

Serves 4

Sauce:
1 cup mayonnaise
¼ cup mint leaves, chopped
1 garlic clove, minced
1 tablespoon lemon juice
Salt and pepper to taste

In a small bowl, mix the mayonnaise with the mint, garlic, and lemon juice. Season with salt and pepper, then refrigerate.

Lamb burgers:
2 to 3 tablespoons dried currants
2 to 3 tablespoons pine nuts
2 tablespoons flat-leaf parsley, coarsely chopped
1 to 2 teaspoons lemon zest, finely grated
½ teaspoon ground cumin
½ teaspoon ground coriander
½ teaspoon cinnamon
1 teaspoon lemon juice
1 teaspoon salt
1¾ pounds lamb, freshly ground
Vegetable oil for the grill
4 hamburger buns or Kaiser rolls

In a mini-food processor, combine the dried currants, pine nuts, chopped parsley, lemon zest, cumin, coriander, and cinnamon with the lemon juice and 1 teaspoon salt. Process until a paste forms. Scrape the mixture into a bowl and add the ground lamb.

Using your hands, gently mix the ground meat mixture thoroughly with the seasonings and pat into 4 plump burgers. Set the burgers on a plate, cover them with plastic wrap, and refrigerate for 15 minutes.

Light a grill. Lightly brush the grate with oil. Grill the burgers over a medium-hot fire for 6 minutes per side for medium rare. Grill the buns, cut-side down, until toasted. Set the burgers on the buns and serve with the sauce.

EASY LAMB SHANKS

Barbara Sulman

4 servings

4 lamb shanks
1/4 cup flour
1 teaspoon salt
1 teaspoon pepper
1 teaspoon garlic powder
3 tablespoons olive oil
6 cloves garlic, crushed
1 medium onion, chopped
2 carrots, chopped
1 8-ounce can tomato sauce
1 14-ounce can chicken broth
1/2 cup red wine
1/3 cup red wine vinegar
1 tablespoon sugar
1/8 cup fresh thyme, chopped
1/2 teaspoon dried oregano

Preheat the oven to 350°.

Dredge the lamb shanks in the flour, salt, pepper, and garlic powder.

Heat 2 to 3 tablespoons of olive oil and sear lamb shanks until brown, remove from the pan, and place in a baking casserole dish fitted with a lid.

In the same pan as the meat, sauté the garlic, onion, and carrots until soft, adding additional olive oil if necessary. Combine the tomato sauce, chicken broth, red wine, red wine vinegar, sugar, thyme, and oregano to make a sauce.

Pour sauce over the lamb shanks and bake for 3½ to 4 hours, until very tender.

"Recipes are revered for the memories they evoke as well as for the yummy food created by using them.

"When Michel and I got married almost 50 years ago, I had never cooked a thing, nor did I care to! I had hardly ever turned on a stove, much less turned on a broiler at 19 years of age. My first meal as a new bride was going to be broiled lamb chops, baked potatoes, and a green salad. I do not remember much about the tossed green salad, but the lamp chops caught on fire and the baked potatoes were undercooked and impossible to cut, let alone eat. And that was the beginning of my culinary career.
Thanks to my very strong-stomached, supportive husband, my inspirational mother and grandmother, and my mother-in-law, a legendary baker, I developed a passion for cooking and a love of collecting recipes.

"Although I do not take the time to cook so much anymore, I do love recipes, and as they say, there is always room for one more good one! The Jewish holidays are my favorite time to cook, as they remind me of warm, loving times of eating and hearing about what it took to prepare the meals. I have kept copious records of all the meals I have prepared for company over the years and who came to eat with us. I treasure these records in my file box as they bring back memories of treasured family, friends, and fabulous food."

~ Bobbie Stern

KENNY'S LAMB

Kenny Alhadeff

"Comfort food is what comes to mind when I think of this lamb dish. It is one of my favorites, and I prefer it slathered in ketchup."

Serves 4

2 to 3 pounds lamb shoulder steaks
2 onions, sliced
3 to 4 potatoes, unpeeled and sliced
1 teaspoon salt
1 teaspoon pepper
1 teaspoon garlic powder
1 tablespoon paprika

Preheat the oven to 450°.

Arrange the lamb steaks on the bottom of a 9x13-inch glass dish. Season the lamb with one-third of the salt, pepper, garlic powder, and paprika.

Cover the lamb with the sliced onion and season with one-third of the spices. Cover the onions with the potatoes and sprinkle with the remaining spices. Bake uncovered for 1 hour.

CHICKEN PATTIES (CHICKEN CLOUCHETTE)

Janice & Steve Lewis and Cindy & Gary Stratiner

"This is a family favorite and has been served at many a family dinner. Zara Tarshis, would go to her daughter's home, Joyce Stratiner's, and make many clouchette to ensure enough for dinner and leftovers. She would sometimes make it for Passover Seder substituting the challah with matzo. Zara had been taught most of her famous recipes from her grandmother in Russia when she was a young girl. Her grandmother would sit her on a stool and expect her to watch and learn. Boy, did she ever learn how to cook! It was a joy for her to cook for her family and for many friends in the community. Everything was delicious. Trying to learn from Bubba Zara was always tricky – she cooked by feel and taste. She used to want us to taste the raw fish concoction before we put the gefilte fish balls in the stock. She wanted us to make sure they were the right consistency and had enough pepper. Zara never got sick and lived to the ripe old age of 100, almost 101. She is deeply missed but not forgotten."

Makes 6 to 8 patties

2 whole chicken breasts, ground
2 slices of challah, no crusts, moistened with liquid squeezed out
2 to 3 eggs (depending on size of eggs and chicken breasts)
1 teaspoon salt
1 teaspoon white pepper
1 tablespoon onion powder
1 tablespoon garlic powder
1 chicken bouillon cube
2 tablespoons oil

Preheat the oven to 325°.

Mix together the ground chicken, moistened challah, eggs, salt, white pepper, onion powder, and garlic powder.

Mash the bouillon cube and blend with the oil in a small bowl, and then heat in a large skillet.

With a large spoon, drop the chicken mixture into the pan, slightly flatten, and brown on each side at a medium to high setting. Drain on a paper towel and finish off in the oven for 15 minutes.

TIPS & TRICKS:

- You can also fry the patties at a lower temperature until they are cooked through.

LEMON CHICKEN MILANESE

Michelle Sloan

Serves 4

4 boneless, skinless chicken breast halves
2 large eggs
1¼ cups panko breadcrumbs
3 tablespoons fresh parsley, chopped
2 teaspoons fresh oregano, chopped
1 teaspoon kosher salt
¾ teaspoon ground black pepper
4 tablespoons olive oil
2 tablespoons fresh lemon juice

Using a rolling pin, between sheets of plastic flatten chicken breasts to ½-inch thick.

Whisk the eggs in a medium bowl to blend.

Mix the Panko breadcrumbs, 2 tablespoons of the parsley, oregano, and salt and pepper in a pie plate.

Dip chicken in the beaten eggs and turn to coat. Dredge in the breadcrumb mixture, coating completely.

Heat 3 tablespoons of the oil in large nonstick skillet over medium heat. Add chicken and sauté until golden brown and cooked through, about 5 minutes per side.

Transfer chicken to plates, sprinkle with the remaining parsley and lemon juice.

TIPS & TRICKS:

- Serve arugula salad dressed with a lemon vinaigrette on top of the chicken.
- Tomato bruschetta also complements this dish very well.

STIR-FRY CHICKEN

Barbara Sulman

"A delicious, healthy, and easy dinner; very satisfying and no need to go out for Sunday Chinese! Our kids always love this dish, and I was able to add vegetables according to their preferences. We loved the sauce, so I often make extra for the rice."

Serves 2 to 3

1 tablespoon corn starch
5 tablespoons soy sauce, divided
1 pound boneless, skinless chicken breasts, cubed
1 tablespoon dry sherry
2 teaspoons sugar
1 teaspoon vinegar
¼ cup oil
1 medium onion, sliced
1 medium red or green pepper, sliced
1 cup broccoli florets (or any vegetable of your choice)
1 cup bean sprouts

Combine the cornstarch and 1 tablespoon of the soy sauce in a bowl, add the chicken, and stir to coat. Set aside.

In a separate bowl, combine the remaining soy sauce, sherry, sugar, and vinegar. Set aside.

Heat the oil in a wok, add the chicken, and cook for 2 to 3 minutes. Remove the chicken mixture from the wok. Set aside.

Add the onion, red or green pepper, and broccoli to the wok, and stir-fry until brown and crisp, 3 to 5 minutes.

Return the chicken to the wok with the vegetables, cook another 2 to 3 minutes until tender, stirring constantly. Add the bean sprouts.

Pour the soy sauce mixture into the wok, stir, cover, and cook for about 1 minute.

Serve over white or brown rice.

BEER CAN CHICKEN

Jordan Lott

"This is a fun and unique way to barbecue chicken."

Serves 4

1 four-pound whole chicken
1 can of light beer
½ lime
3 to 4 tablespoons spice rub

Spice Rub:
1 pound Cajun seasoning (such as McCormick Cajun Seasoning)
¼ cup fennel seed
¼ cup coriander seed
¼ cup sesame seeds
2 tablespoons dried thyme
2 tablespoons dried oregano
2 tablespoons smoked paprika
¼ teaspoon Coleman's dry mustard powder
¼ teaspoon tumeric
¼ teaspoon celery seed

Toast all seeds until fragrant. Allow to cool for 5 to 10 minutes, then grind in a spice/coffee grinder. (You may skip this step if you would like, but the grinding does enhance the flavor of the rub.) Add additional spices to the Cajun seasoning if desired.

Clean, dry, and rub the chicken with spice blend. Let sit 20 to 30 minutes before you begin grilling.

Place a large sheet of aluminum foil on the grill, then place the beer can chicken holder on top. Open and pour out (or drink) about 3 ounces from the can of beer, then place it in holder. Place chicken, cavity down, over the can and holder and pin wings back so they don't burn. If you don't have a beer can chicken holder, stuff the chicken with the beer can before placing it on the grill and balance the chicken, using the legs as a tripod.

Squeeze lime juice into the neck of the chicken, and use the rind to cork the neck, trapping in the moisture.

TIPS & TRICKS:

- When you are ready to rub on the spice mixture, spoon what you need into a separate little bowl. Spoon more if necessary, but do not touch the remaining rub mixture with fingers that have touched the chicken, to prevent contamination.
- This recipe will make enough spice rub for 4 chickens, so store what you do not use in an air-tight container in a cool dry place.

Grill over low to medium heat for about 1 hour and 15 minutes or until the chicken reads 180°F. Turn off the grill and move the chicken to a cutting board. (The beer can will be hot, so be careful.) Cover the chicken loosely with aluminum foil and let rest 10 minutes before carving.

If using a gas grill, do NOT turn the grill on before the chicken is situated. Secure the foil and place the beer and chicken on a cold grill.

GRANDPA'S ROAST CHICKEN

Craig Sternberg

"I don't cook, but, on two occasions, I did take a cooking class at Herzl-Ner Tamid called, 'Men Cooking for Shabbat.' The course taught us a lot more than just cooking! We learned traditions and the importance of food preparation and religious observance."

Serves 4 to 6

1 3- to 4-pound chicken, quartered
1 medium onion
¼ teaspoon black pepper
¼ teaspoon chili powder
Salt to taste
1 heaping teaspoon whole dry rosemary
1 heaping tablespoon paprika
2 pounds Yukon Gold potatoes, unpeeled, washed, and trimmed of "eyes"
1 tablespoon olive oil

Preheat the oven to 375°. Remove any feathers and excess fat from the chicken. Wash the chicken and pat dry.

Slice the onion and place it on the bottom of the roasting pan.

Mix the pepper, chili powder, salt, rosemary, and paprika, and season the chicken with three-quarters of the mixture.

Quarter the potatoes and toss them with the olive oil. Sprinkle them with the remaining spice mixture and add them to the roasting pan.

Bake the chicken, skin-side up, for 50 to 60 minutes, occasionally basting with the pan juices.

BAKED LEMON CHICKEN

Cynthia Shifrin

"One night while having Shabbat dinner at my friend Debra Rettman's, she served a chicken dish that was so scrumptious I couldn't stop tasting it. I was intrigued that even though it appeared to be just ordinary plain chicken, it tasted anything but ordinary or plain. After my third helping, I asked her what she did to make it taste so delish. She shared with me that one of the things she did was stuff the cavity with a whole lemon cut in half – something I had often done, yet my chicken didn't have that same delectable flavor. As she went on further, she said after it's done baking, she squeezes the juice from the baked lemon over the chicken...bingo! That was an important step I hadn't done, and doing so makes such a difference. Debra also rubs fresh garlic over the chicken before baking and uses just pepper as a spice. In my version, I use the prepared crushed garlic in a jar that has almost a paste-like consistency and found it actually works better than the chopped kind.

"Here's my own recipe that was inspired by Debra Rettman's delectable baked chicken."

Serves 4 to 5

1 whole chicken, about 5 to 5½ pounds
2 large lemons
1 tablespoon paprika
1 tablespoon ground coriander
1 tablespoon curry powder
1 teaspoon kosher salt
Freshly ground pepper to taste
2 tablespoons olive oil
2 tablespoons garlic, crushed (not chopped)
1 cup white wine
½ cup water

Preheat the oven to 425° with the rack placed in the lower third of the oven.

Under cold water, thoroughly rinse the outside and inside of the chicken and pat dry.

In a small bowl, make a wet rub with the paprika, coriander, curry powder, salt, pepper, olive oil, and crushed garlic, then liberally rub it over the entire outside and inside of the chicken. Cut the two lemons in half and stuff them into the chicken cavity. If you don't have room for one of the halves, place it in the opening at the neck and secure it closed with a toothpick.

Place the chicken breast-side down on a rack set in a roasting pan. Pour the white wine and water into the bottom of the pan. (Periodically, you might need to add extra water, as the liquid evaporates during the cooking process.)

Bake for 35 minutes, then carefully turn the chicken over (using two large meat forks with one in the neck and one in the cavity) and bake breast-side up for an additional 30 to 35 minutes, or until a meat thermometer reads 165° (do not touch the bone). Remove from the oven and allow the chicken to rest for at least 5 to 10 minutes before cutting, allowing the juices to drip down through the meat. Just before serving, squeeze the juice from the baked lemon over the chicken.

SALLY'S FRIDAY NIGHT CHICKEN

Roz Poll

"My mother-in-law always served her chicken with asparagus, noodle kugel, and a wonderful, big salad with lots of cucumbers, radishes, and tomatoes. The spices were never measured, just liberally sprinkled on the chicken."

Serves 4 to 6

1 chicken, cut into serving pieces with skin and bones
½ tablespoon olive oil (optional)
2 teaspoons garlic powder
2 teaspoons salt-free seasoning blend
1 teaspoon sweet paprika
1 teaspoon salt

Preheat the oven to 350°.

Wash the chicken and pat dry.

On a foil-lined, rimmed baking sheet, place the chicken skin-side down. If desired, brush with ¼ tablespoon of the olive oil.

In a small bowl, combine the garlic powder, salt-free seasoning, paprika, and salt. Sprinkle the chicken liberally with the mixture.

Increase the oven to broil and place the chicken under the broiler until it becomes quite brown. Remove the chicken from the oven and flip the pieces over, brushing with remaining olive oil, if desired. Season the chicken with the other half of the seasoning mixture and broil again until nicely browned.

Remove the chicken from the oven, move the rack to the middle of the oven, and reduce the oven temperature to 350°. Return the chicken back to the oven and bake uncovered for approximately 45 minutes.

ROASTED CHICKEN WITH LEMON, GARLIC, AND OREGANO

Gail Alexander

Serves 12

1/4 cup fresh lemon juice
1/4 cup fresh oregano, finely chopped
2 tablespoons garlic, minced
2 tablespoons kosher salt
2 teaspoons black pepper
1/3 cup olive oil
12 chicken legs, rinsed and dried
8 chicken breasts, rinsed and dried
5 lemons, cut into 1/3-inch slices

Whisk together the lemon juice, oregano, garlic, ½ tablespoon of the salt, and ½ teaspoon of the pepper in a large bowl. Pour the oil in a slow and steady stream, whisking constantly.

Season the chicken with the remaining 1½ tablespoons of salt and 1½ teaspoons of pepper, then place the seasoned chicken in two large plastic bags. Add the marinade equally over the chicken in each bag and marinate for at least a few hours (or overnight), turning the chicken to cover with the marinade.

Preheat the oven to 500°.

Remove the chicken from the bag and lay the pieces in two shallow pans in the upper and lower thirds of the oven. Bake for 40 minutes, rotating the pans halfway through the cooking time. When finished, the skin should be crisp.

Place the chicken pieces on a large platter and garnish with lemon slices.

PAPRIKA CHICKEN

Judy Schocken

Serves 4 to 6

2 tablespoons vegetable oil
1 large onion, diced
1 chicken, cut into pieces
1 green pepper, sliced
1 14½-ounce can tomatoes
¾ cup cold water
3 tablespoons paprika (try Hungarian Sweet paprika)
Salt and pepper, to taste
2 tablespoons flour

In a large ovenproof sauté pan with a lid, sauté the onions in the oil over medium heat. When golden brown, remove from the pan and use that oil to brown the chicken pieces.

Place the sautéed onions back in the pan with the chicken and add the sliced green pepper, tomatoes, ¼ cup of the water, paprika, salt, and pepper. Cover and simmer for 1½ to 2 hours.

Place ½ cup of the water in a small jar with lid and add the flour. Shake well. Using a strainer, add the mixture to the chicken and stir.

Cook for an additional 10 minutes to thicken the sauce. Serve with noodles, potatoes, dumplings, or sauerkraut.

ORANGE-GLAZED CHICKEN

Bernice Rind

Makes 4 servings

1 chicken, 2 ½ to 3 pounds, cut into pieces
1 6-ounce can frozen orange juice, thawed
2 tablespoons candied ginger, slivered
¼ teaspoon pepper
¼ cup water
1 clove garlic, crushed
2 tablespoons soy sauce
1 teaspoon salt (optional)

Place the chicken pieces in a shallow dish. In a medium bowl, combine the orange juice, candied ginger, pepper, water, garlic, soy sauce, and salt, and pour the mixture over the chicken. Cover and marinate the chicken in the refrigerator for at least 3 hours (or overnight), turning the pieces occasionally.

Preheat the oven to 350°. Move the chicken to a roasting pan, reserving the marinade. Bake the chicken for 45 minutes, basting occasionally with the reserved marinade.

MILDRED ROSENBAUM'S CHICKEN TERIYAKI

Betsy Schneier

"Mildred Hardin Rosenbaum, my mother and co-founder of WSJHS, grew up in a strictly observant Orthodox household. Due to a childhood accident, she became independent at an early age and left home in her teens to pursue graduate school in New York. There she met and married her husband, Dr. Harold Rosenbaum. In 1953, after his military service, always curious to pursue 'interesting' life experiences, she and my father decided to move to Seattle, where he became a well-known pediatric dentist.

"Dad's office was just across the street from the University of Washington campus. Soon my parents began hosting foreign students from all over the world, becoming surrogate parents for forty-two young people. Some lived with us while I was growing up, including a series of young women from Taiwan and Japan. To this day, Mother keeps in touch with over half of them!

"My parents entertained frequently. Mom never thought much of her own mother's culinary skills, and she liked to come up with exotic recipes, so she gathered new recipes

by talking to her students and consulting books. This recipe was her favorite. I suspect she blended instructions from several sources, but the taste never ceased to elicit compliments from guests.

"When I entertained my new father-in-law for the very first time, my anxiety was compounded by lack of time to prepare for his visit due to professional obligations. So I turned to this recipe, figuring that it would be easy because of its familiarity. Alas, I forgot to discard the marinade before grilling the chicken, so the meal was inedible – but good sport that he was, Jason's late father was kind enough to ask for seconds!"

Makes 4 servings

1 cup soy sauce
½ cup sugar
1 clove garlic, crushed
¼ teaspoon ground ginger
3 pounds chicken, cut into eight pieces
Salt and pepper to taste
Oil to coat chicken
1 cup canned pineapple chunks, with juice
1 green pepper, sliced
1 medium onion, sliced

Mix the soy, sugar, garlic, and ground ginger in a bowl. Put the chicken in a large dish in a single layer, and pour the marinade over the chicken. Cover the dish and marinate the chicken in the refrigerator for several hours, or overnight if possible.

Preheat the oven to 350° (or 330° if you are using a convection oven). Put the chicken in a baking pan, reserving the marinade for later use. Brush the chicken with oil and season it to taste with salt and pepper.

Roast the chicken for about 30 minutes. Turn the pieces over and add the pineapple, pineapple juice, green pepper, and onion to the pan. Roast the chicken another 30 to 40 minutes, basting with the marinade every 10 minutes.

TIPS & TRICKS:

- ❖ If the chicken browns too quickly, you can cover the pan with foil.

CHICKEN WITH FENNEL, FIGS, AND NORTH AFRICAN SPICES

Brooke Benaroya Dickson

Serves 8

8 chicken legs, whole or thighs and drumsticks separated
OR 2 chickens cut into 8 pieces
3 tablespoons olive oil
1 onion, finely chopped
2 fennel bulbs, finely chopped
4 cloves garlic, minced
3 tablespoons fennel seeds, ground
2 tablespoons coriander, ground
1 star anise, ground
4 cloves, ground
2 tablespoons black mustard seeds
2 tablespoons *ras el hanout* (See TIPS AND TRICKS)
Pinch to 1 teaspoon chili powder
1 cup white wine
1½ to 2 cups chicken stock
Zest of one orange (optional)
10 to 20 figs, chopped
1 tablespoon honey (optional if the figs are not perfectly ripe)

TIPS & TRICKS:

- When fresh figs are not in season, add chopped dried figs with the wine. Or, for an equally delicious dish, substitute a can of drained chopped tomatoes for the figs.
- *Ras el hanout* is a North African blend of twenty spices or more. It is available at Market Spice in the Pike Place Market.

Heat a heavy-bottomed pan over medium heat and add the oil until it is quite hot. In batches, add chicken pieces skin-side down, then turn and brown on all sides, about 12 minutes. Set browned pieces aside and pour off all but 1 or 2 tablespoons of the fat.

Add the onions and fennel in the remaining fat and cook until translucent, about 5 minutes.

In a separate pan, toast fennel and coriander. Grind fennel, coriander, star anise, and cloves with a mortar and pestle.

Combine the garlic, ground fennel, coriander, star anise, and cloves, with the black mustard seeds, ras el hanout, and chili powder, season with salt and pepper, and cook 1 to 2 minutes. Add wine, deglaze the pan, reduce the wine for a minute or two, then add the orange zest. Set aside.

Pack the chicken tightly into a baking dish in a single layer, skin-side up. Pour over the spice mixture and pack it into the chicken. Sprinkle zest and figs, and drizzle optional honey over the top. Pour chicken stock over to nearly cover. Cover and refrigerate 24 hours or longer.

Preheat the oven to 325°.

Remove the chicken from the refrigerator and let it sit at room temperature for 30 minutes. Cook the chicken for about 45 minutes, until the sauce is simmering. Taste and adjust seasoning. The chicken can be served right out of the baking dish or removed to a serving platter. Reduce the cooking liquid over high heat then pour over the chicken.

MEDITERRANEAN CHICKEN

Inez Caspi

"I always need an easy and delicious chicken dish for the holidays or Shabbat. I love the olives, which remind our family of the many years we lived in Israel."

Serves 6

1 roasting chicken, cut into pieces
1 clove garlic, peeled and chopped
Salt and pepper
Paprika
Italian herbs
2 tablespoons olive oil
1 onion, thinly sliced
1 pound peppers, mixed colors, cut into strips
1 pound tomatoes, skinned and chopped
¾ cup pitted black olives

Rub the chicken pieces with the garlic and season with the salt, pepper, paprika, and Italian herbs.

Heat the oil in a heavy pot and brown the chicken pieces on all sides. Remove the chicken and lay it on a plate. Lower the heat, add the onions, and cook until golden and soft. Add the peppers and tomatoes, and cook for 5 minutes.

Return the chicken pieces to the pot and layer on the vegetables. Season to taste and cover. Cook the chicken on medium heat for 50 to 60 minutes or until tender. Add the olives to pot after the chicken is tender and heat for another few minutes.

Fish: Sweet 'n Sour, Smoked 'n Steamed, Stuffed 'n Sauced

The Jewish relationship to fish doesn't begin with a bagel, a shmear, and a pile of smoked salmon or a slice of rye with a baseball-sized mound of tuna. Even the seemingly archaic bottles of briny gefilte fish are the legacy of thousands of years of aquatic culinary development.

The story begins with the Torah, which permits only fish with fins and scales for consumption. Thus this ancient code is integral to what became Jewish culinary heritage. Fish became a customary dish on the Sabbath presumably for economic reasons, but also for spiritual reasons: In the creation account of Genesis, God blesses the fifth, sixth and seventh days, which correspond to the creation of fish, humans, and the Sabbath. In folklore, fish has also stood for fertility, luck, and even the messianic era!

Geography is as important as religious guidelines and customs. The geographical, cultural, and economic influences experienced by Jewish communities throughout time and across the world tell subtle stories through food. These factors led to that Jewish spirit of creativity in the kitchen, and from them the most popular form of Jewish fish, the gefilte, was born. It may be hard to think of gefilte fish as ingenious rather than a lump of slimy gray matter redeemed only by horseradish. But this matriarch of Eastern European Jewish fish recipes began as a way to utilize the region's available offerings and circumvent the rabbinic restriction of separating bones from fish on Shabbat.

We received many gefilte fish recipes, with strong memories attached. Jerry Cone can still recall the aroma of simmering fish balls from nearly 75 years ago, and Pip Meyerson remembers the scent of his mother's gefilte fish permeating the neighborhood after she lost her sense of smell. Others, like "Bubbe" Gitel innovated the recipe with locally available salmon, while Mary Noble remains a purist to the ingredients her mother, a Holocaust survivor, swore by. As the recipe for this "stuffed fish" has traveled from country to country and person to person, it has taken on new flavors, techniques, and to no small extent rival loyalties. And it's not stuffed anymore either, which says something about change.

The other fish recipes in this chapter highlight the abundance of fresh salmon in the Northwest. Nearly all of the recipes and stories, Ashkenazi and Sephardic alike, call for salmon – either mixed into gefilte fish, in Sheila Sternberg's steamed salmon, dressed with Turkish plums, or in the *pescado con huevos y limon*. What we're left with is, as the Torah suggests, a blessing of creation.

TIDBIT:

It is not permitted to pick bones out of fish on Shabbat, a time when fish is customarily served. *Borer*, or choosing, is one of the 39 types of work prohibited on Shabbat. Thus Eastern European Jewish cooks prepared ground "gefilte" fish for Shabbat meals.

"Fish and Fishing." *Encyclopedia Judaica* (1972).

Claudia Roden. "Gefilte Fish and the Jews." *Jewish Heritage Online Magazine.*

FISH: SWEET 'N SOUR, SMOKED 'N STEAMED, STUFFED 'N SAUCED

GITEL'S SWEET AND SOUR FISH

Cindy Muscatel, Mimi Sorkin, Rabbi Lennard Thal, and Bonnie Zell

"'When Bubbe Gitel arrived in Seattle on the train from Bellingham, she reminded us all of Mary Poppins,' her granddaughter, Cindy Muscatel recalls. 'I still remember standing there in the terminal with my dad, waiting for her and my grandfather. She always carried a huge, black satchel. When we'd get home, Bubbe Gitel would pull goodie after homemade goodie out of its depths. First there'd be the baked goods – maybe on this trip cinnamon rolls, bagels, a pie, or her famous cookies (that no one ever got the recipe for). Next, she'd retrieve the mainstays – chopped liver, kreplach in chicken soup, borscht, gefilte fish, or her amazing sweet and sour salmon...you name it! How it all fit in that satchel still is a mystery.'

"Gertrude (Gitel) Thal's gefilte fish was legendary in Bellingham, Washington. Often, she was given free salmon to make her all-salmon gefilte fish just so the fish monger could have a sample for himself.

"Gitel was such a consummate cook that she never measured the amount of her ingredients. If you asked, she'd say 'a half eggshell of this or a handful of that, a little of this and a little of that.'

"'I started shadowing her and measuring her handfuls,' Cindy says. 'But I still use recipes that call for half an eggshell of something.'

"Years ago, Gitel's sister-in-law, Rose, went over to watch Gitel prepare the famous fish delicacies. Rose, too, quantified every little bit of this and that into recipes. That's why today we are able to make not only Gitel's gefilte fish, but also her even more delicious sweet and sour salmon."

Serves 10-12

3 pounds salmon, 1-inch thick, cut into chunks
2 large onions, left whole
1 cup cider vinegar
1 cup sugar
½ tablespoon whole allspice
¼ cup raisins
½ cup brown sugar
Salt and pepper, to taste

Boil 1 quart of water in a medium pot and add the onions. Cook the onions until they are tender. Remove them from the water, reserving the water, and purée. Return the puréed onions to the reserved liquid.

Add the cider vinegar, white sugar, allspice, raisins, brown sugar, salt and pepper. Bring everything to a boil and add the fish piece by piece. Boil for 15 minutes.

Let the fish cool in the pot, slightly covered. When cooled, place the fish in a storage container and strain the poaching liquid through a sieve into the container. Serve cold.

MOM'S SWEET AND SOUR FISH

Helen Stusser

"This recipe was passed down to my mother, Marion Rosen, by her mother, Helen Blumenthal, and then to me. It was usually served on Passover, but it also showed up at other family celebrations."

4 pieces salmon (4 to 6 ounces each)
1 lemon, sliced
1 onion, sliced
1 cup raisins

Sauce:
7 ginger snaps, crushed
2 tablespoons vinegar
½ cup maple syrup
½ cup brown sugar
½ cup slivered almonds

Place the salmon in a shallow frying pan and add just enough water to cover the fish. Add the lemon slices, onion slices, and the raisins. Boil until "just nice" – 5 to 6 minutes or until done. Remove the fish and drain it on paper towels. Do not discard the cooking liquid. Keep the fish warm on a serving platter.

Add the ginger snaps, vinegar, maple syrup, brown sugar, and almonds to the water the fish was cooked in. Boil the sauce until it is thickened. Pour the sauce over the salmon before serving.

MARGARET SCHNEIDERMAN'S PICKLED FISH

Judy Rosen

"This is something my late mother-in-law served at every Jewish holiday, every brunch, and every dinner party."

Serves 12 to 16

1½ pounds onions, sliced
4 pounds salmon, skinned, cut into large cubes
2 14-ounce bottles ketchup
1 24-ounce jar sliced cucumber chips, drained, brine reserved, chopped

Layer in a Dutch oven as follows:

½ of the sliced onions
½ of the salmon
1 bottle of the ketchup
½ jar of the chopped pickles

Repeat layers. Pour the reserved cucumber chip brine over the layers.

Bring the fish to a careful boil, then simmer. Cook, covered, 30 to 40 minutes. Serve the fish cold or at room temperature.

SMOKED SALMON

Barrie Galanti

"I originally got this recipe from my parents, Ruth and Al Sanft. The process takes almost 24 hours, but it is worth the wait."

Serves 20

5 pounds salmon, filleted, deboned, and cut into 6 pieces
30 cups cold water
1½ cups rock salt
1 cup brown sugar
Garlic powder, onion powder, and freshly ground pepper, for sprinkling

To brine the salmon, mix the cold water, salt, and brown sugar together in a large pot. Add the fish, using heavy plates to keep the fish completely submerged. Leave the fish in the water for 8 hours.

Take the fish out of the brine one piece at a time, rinse in cold water, and pat each piece dry. Lay the fish out on racks (oven racks or cooling racks) and dry for at least 6 to 8 hours.

Prepare the fish for smoking by setting the dry fish on smoker racks, season it with the garlic powder, onion powder, and pepper. Set the smoking chips in the bottom of the smoker, being sure you add more chips at least once while the fish is cooking. Make sure there is a constant stream of smoke. Smoke the fish for 4 to 6 hours until the fish is firm, but not dry.

Once the salmon is smoked, cool it on racks on a counter. If the salmon is not cooled, it will fall apart. Salmon is done when it looks cooked and has milky striations on top.

When it is done and cooled, wrap the pieces of salmon in waxed paper, followed by a layer of foil, then refrigerate.

TIPS & TRICKS:

❖ Our schedule for making the fish is as follows: brine overnight; dry early in the morning; and start smoking by the afternoon.

> *"Piscado con Avramila (fish with sour plum sauce) was handed down within my family from generation to generation. The fabulous climate of Turkey begot the most fabulous plums. The cities from which most of us originated (Istanbul, Ismir, Tekirdag, all port cities) also offered an abundance of meaty fish. Picture yourself enjoying this dish with a glass of raki, overlooking the tremendous view of the Bosphorous Strait with good company, and Turkish music in the background."*
>
> ~ Janti Baroh

SALMON WITH TOMATO SAUCE

Doreen Alhadeff

"My dad, Cookie Cohen, worked for decades at Pure Food Fish at the Pike Place Market. Not only was he was a friendly and welcome face to his customers who truly enjoyed and counted on listening to his wonderful stories and jokes, he was also appreciated for the fish he would select for them. Dad's customers always knew they could rely on him for the freshest catch. The following recipe is a Cohen and Alhadeff family staple."

Serves 6

1½ pounds salmon, cut into individual servings
¾ teaspoon salt
2 tablespoons olive oil
2 medium onions, halved then sliced
1½ lemons, juiced
2 15-ounce cans diced tomatoes in purée
1 8-ounce can tomato sauce
Handful of fresh parsley, chopped

Season the salmon with ¼ teaspoon of the salt.

Cook the onions in olive oil until almost soft. Add the tomatoes and tomato sauce to the onions and cook over low heat for 30 to 40 minutes. Add the lemon juice, the remaining ½ teaspoon of the salt, and cook another 20 minutes. Taste to see if it needs more lemon.

Preheat the oven to 325°.

Put the tomato mixture in the bottom of a 9x13-inch baking dish. Place the salmon pieces on top of the mixture, spooning a bit of the sauce over the fish.

TIPS & TRICKS:

❖ If cooling before serving, be sure the foil is off the pan.

Cover with foil and bake for 45 minutes, shaking the pan at least once during baking. Remove from the oven and uncover. Transfer the salmon pieces to a serving dish and spoon the tomato mixture over it. Sprinkle with the parsley and serve immediately or cool slightly.

PESCADO CON HUEVOS Y LIMON (FISH WITH EGG AND LEMON SAUCE)

Kathie Barokas

"When I was first married, my mother-in-law always prepared fish with lemon sauce. It was served cold, as a first course, right after the blessings, usually at holiday meals such as Rosh Hashanah and Passover. It makes a beautiful dish with its delicious lemon and egg sauce."

Serves 6 to 10

3 to 4 pounds salmon
1 teaspoon salt, or more to taste
3 to 4 tablespoons parsley, chopped
1 tablespoon canola oil
3 medium lemons, juiced (about ¾ cup)
5 eggs, room temperature, beaten

Cut the fish into serving portions approximately ¼ pound each. Using a 12-inch high-sided frying pan just large enough to accommodate the fish in one layer, add enough water to barely reach the top of the fish. Add the salt, 2 tablespoons of the parsley, oil, and 1 tablespoon lemon juice and bring to a boil. Add the fish and cook until tender, about 5 to 10 minutes. Remove the fish from the heat. Reserve the poaching liquid.

In a separate bowl, beat the eggs and remaining lemon juice. Add ½ cup of the poaching liquid, only a few tablespoons at a time, to the egg mixture. Put the egg mixture back into the fish pan and continue to cook at a very low heat, shaking the pan until the sauce is thickened, another 6 minutes. Don't let the sauce boil.

Carefully transfer the fish to a glass dish. Pour the sauce over the fish, cool, then refrigerate, covered with plastic wrap, until ready to serve. Sprinkle with the remaining parsley.

TIPS & TRICKS:

- ❖ When adding the poaching liquid to the egg mixture, be sure to do it gradually. Otherwise, the sauce will curdle.
- ❖ If using a 10-inch pan, reduce the quantities to 3 eggs and 2 lemons.

It's a ball, it's a patty, it's a loaf...it's...it's gefilte fish!

The ingredients and preparation of gefilte fish vary from family to family no matter the presentation. Traditions surrounding gefilte fish differ from kitchen to kitchen, region to region, and holiday to holiday. Sweet is usually preferred by people of Polish heritage, while savory is preferred by those of Russian descent. Gefilte fish may be served shaped in balls, sliced from a loaf, or formed into patties. It may be poached in fish stock, oven baked, or coated in matzo meal and fried. All is left to individual interpretation and preference.

The ground fish mixture is influenced by regional availability. According to Joey Alhadeff, who worked for his family's fish business and then for Quality Food Centers (QFC), the first QFC to have a specific fish department was the store in University Village in Seattle. The man in charge there at the time, Isaac Scharhon, created a mix of white fish that is still used across the chain's many stores in the Pacific Northwest. It is a blend of carp, a fresh water fish, and snapper, lingcod, and black cod, all salt water fish. Salmon is rarely used in gefilte fish made by anyone from the Midwest, or the East Coast or, for that matter, from the "old country." It is only here in our part of the world that salmon, because of its abundance, is used all on its own or combined with other white fish to make gefilte fish. This is a perfect example of Jews adapting their traditional dishes to the regions in which they find themselves living.

There is one thing and one thing only that people agree on when it comes to gefilte fish. Everyone who makes gefilte fish proudly proclaims their recipe is *the best.* While that may be something all gefilte fish makers have in common, it means no two people ever agree on a recipe that is universally appreciated or accepted. The reason we have included 7 different gefilte fish recipes is because one fact never changes: there is a certain pride to every family's particular way of making gefilte fish.

GEFILTE FISH THE EASY WAY

Ann Neider

"The simple way of making gefilte fish for anybody who is not a food purist."

Serves 8

1 to 2 onions, skins reserved and sliced
1 jar of unsweetened gefilte fish, including the broth
1 carrot, peeled and sliced into ¼-inch pieces
Parsley, as a garnish
Horseradish, for serving

Brown the onion slices in a little oil until limp and golden in color. In the bottom of a large pot, place the onion skins, onions, and carrots. Pour the contents of the gefilte fish jar into the pot. Cover, simmer for about 20 minutes, then cool and refrigerate. When ready to serve, garnish each piece of gefilte fish with a sprig of parsley and a slice of carrot. Serve with horseradish.

GRANDMA WEINSTEIN'S GEFILTE FISH

Lee Weinstein

"Although my mother-in-law, Noralee Leopold Weinstein, was not what I'd call an adventurous cook, what she made, she did well, and I consider her to have been one of the best Jewish cooks I have known. This fish recipe was her mother's and is served hot. It uses salmon, since it is readily available in this area."

Makes approximately 80 balls

Stock:
9 onions, chopped
Oil
1 carrot, chopped
2 ribs celery, chopped
Tips and ends from fish (see list below for fish amounts)
Salt
Pepper
Garlic powder

Brown the onions in oil. For the broth, put one-third of the browned onions in a large pot, reserving the remaining two-thirds of the onions for the fish. Add the carrot, celery, and the fish tips and ends to the pot; then add water to cover. Add the salt, pepper, and garlic powder to taste. Bring to a boil, cover, and simmer for 1 hour.

Fish:
3 carrots
2 stalks celery
1 onion, chopped
3 pounds salmon, ground
2 pounds black cod, ground
5 eggs
5 teaspoons salt
Garlic powder
Pepper
3 teaspoons Accent (optional)
2 teaspoons sugar
Matzo meal (about a handful)
Oil, for frying
3 cups water

Grind the carrots, celery, and onion. Add that mixture and the remaining two-thirds of the browned onions to the salmon, cod, and eggs in a large bowl. Add the salt, garlic powder, pepper, Accent, and sugar, and mix well.

Add the matzo meal and water to the mixture until desired consistency is achieved, allowing you to form the mixture into balls. The more water you use, the lighter the balls will be. The dough should be gummy, not stiff.

Heat the oil in an electric fry pan or on the stovetop to 350°.

Keep your hands wet while rolling the balls, to prevent sticking. Form fish balls using 1½ teaspoons of fish mixture each. Fry the balls until brown.

Bring the broth to a boil and add the fish. Cover and boil for 1 hour.

TIPS & TRICKS:

- If you don't have a meat grinder, have the fish ground at the market.
- Recipe can be made ahead and frozen. Freeze fish and broth in separate containers. To serve, heat balls in boiling broth for about 1 hour.

GEFILTE FISH FOR PESACH

Pip and Miriam Meyerson

"Pip's mother lost her sense of smell years ago. So she was oblivious to the strong fishy smell permeating the house and neighborhood when she'd make gefilte fish. Pip would never look forward to coming home from school during those times, but of course loved to eat the delicious gefilte fish, loaded with horseradish."

Makes 15 to 18 balls

Stock:
Fish bones and head (ask for them when ordering fish)
1½ quarts water
3 carrots, sliced
3 stalks celery, chopped
1 onion, diced
1 teaspoon salt
1 teaspoon pepper

Place the fish head and bones in a pot with the water, carrots, celery, onion, salt, and pepper. Cover and boil, over medium heat, while preparing fish.

Fish:
3 pounds fish (1½ pounds white fish and 1½ pounds salmon)
1 onion, finely ground
3 eggs
½ teaspoon salt
¼ teaspoon pepper
¼ cup water
¼ cup matzo meal

Horseradish, for serving

Place the fish into a large mixing bowl. Grind the onion into the fish mixture. Add the eggs, salt, pepper, water, and matzo meal to the fish mixture. Have a bowl of clean water ready, so hands can be moistened to shape the fish mixture into balls, as it is sticky.

Turn the fish stock to low, but keep it boiling. Very carefully, drop the fish balls into the stock. Cover and cook for 1 to 1½ hours. The fish balls should be covered by the stock at all times; add more water if necessary. Remove the carrot slices after cooking. Cool the fish.

To serve place a piece of gefilte fish on lettuce leaf, garnish with a carrot slice, and serve with horseradish.

AUNTIE SYL'S GEFILTE FISH

Cindy Masin

"Every family has a designated gefilte fish maker. In our family, it was my aunt, Sylvia Oseran, who taught me the art of making gefilte fish. She learned from her mother-in-law, Bessie Grief. I'm not sure who Bessie learned from, but Auntie Sylvia saved Bessie's wooden bowl and chopping tool, which she continued to use the two times a year she prepared gefilte fish, Rosh Hashanah and Passover. Auntie Sylvia's recipe called for 9 pounds of fish; 6 were a blend of white fish, and 3 were salmon. On her recipe, Auntie Sylvia notated in several places to 'chop, chop, chop,' as the fish needed to be a certain consistency. When I make it, I use an electric mixer to mix, mix, mix. Sylvia's fish contained barely a handful of matzo meal, but it did contain sugar, a fair amount of it, and it was tinged with flecks of carrots, celery, and sweet onion. She would place the uncooked balls of fish into stock that had been flavored with fish heads and bones, more onions and carrots, and then topped with onion skins. The onion skins colored the fish light brown, a detail not to be overlooked. For years, I made the gefilte fish with Auntie Sylvia, and then I was on my own. Those in our family who weren't particularly fond of the fish 'aroma' for three days after making gefilte fish were very happy when my sister-in-law, Marilyn Kremen, said she would take over as the new designated gefilte fish maker."

Makes 45 to 50 balls

Stock:
8 onions, sliced, reserving the brown skins
8 carrots, peeled and sliced in ¼-inch slices
¼ cup sugar
4 fish heads and skeletons
1 tablespoon salt
1 tablespoon pepper

In each of two very large pots, place 4 onions, 4 carrots, 1/8 cup sugar, 2 fish heads, 2 skeletons, 1/2 tablespoon of the salt and 1/2 tablespoon of the pepper. Add water to reach halfway up the top of each pot. Bring the water to a boil and skim the foam that rises to the top. Continue to boil slowly while chopping the fish.

Fish:
9 pounds of ground fish (6 pounds white fish blend and 3 pounds salmon)
8 carrots, peeled and finely ground
8 stalks celery, finely ground
8 onions, finely ground, reserving the brown skins
6 cups water
1 tablespoon salt
1 tablespoon pepper
4½ cups water

6 eggs, beaten
½ cup matzo meal
4 to 5 drops of Tabasco sauce
¾ to 1 cup sugar
Paprika, for sprinkling

Red horseradish, for serving

Using a hand mixer or electric stand mixer, combine the fish, carrots, celery, and onions, and start mixing. During mixing, stop and add 3 cups of the water, 3 of the eggs, ¼ cup of the matzo meal, ½ tablespoon of the salt, ½ tablespoon of the pepper, a few drops of Tabasco sauce, and a scant ½ cup of the sugar, and mix, mix, mix. Add the remaining water, eggs, matzo meal, salt, pepper, Tabasco sauce, and sugar, and continuing to mix, mix, mix. You can mix the fish in two batches if your bowl is not large enough.

When the fish is sufficiently mixed, dip your hands in cold water and form the fish mixture into balls about the size of a small, oval tennis ball. Carefully drop each ball, as it is formed, into the simmering fish stock, dividing the balls between the two pots. The balls will be on top of one another by the time you are finished forming them.

Sprinkle paprika on top of the fish balls, then cover with the reserved brown onion skins so the skin is touching the gefilte fish. Cover the pots and simmer for 2½ hours, removing the lids for the last 20 minutes.

When done, remove and discard the onion peels and gently and carefully transfer the fish to Pyrex dishes – some of the gefilte fish balls may be stuck together. Strain the poaching liquid into a separate bowl and remove the sliced carrots from the rest of the bones. Spoon some liquid and place the carrots over the fish. Cool then refrigerate. Serve each piece on a lettuce leaf with a carrot on top and a teaspoon of red horseradish on the side.

GRANDMA EVA'S GEFILTE FISH

Sandra Ostroff

"Grandma Eva was the matriarch of our family and a fabulous cook. She was born in Lodz, Poland, and came to Seattle in about 1910 via Galveston, Texas. She hosted our family dinners for years, until she was well into her 80s and was the only one in our family who made the gefilte fish, which is something I love. My mom was about 65 and had no interest in learning how to do it. I realized that if I didn't learn how to make it, the recipe would die with her and be gone forever. Grandma Eva was wonderful cook, and this is one of my favorites. She didn't have a recipe. It was all in her head. I had to watch closely and count and measure everything that was in it, because she did it strictly by texture. The recipe has changed and evolved slightly over the years. I've used different amounts of eggs, and I don't add sugar, but I think she may have. You can try adding 1 teaspoon of sugar per pound of fish, if you want. The recipe is a bit complicated and time consuming, but worth it. It can be made into balls or patties."

Makes 8 balls per pound of fish, 32 balls for this recipe

2 pounds ground salmon
2 pounds ground mixed white fish
2 medium sweet onions
4 medium carrots
8 eggs
Salt and white pepper
¼ cup matzo meal or challah bread crumbs
Ice water
Fish stock, for cooking fish balls (fish heads, bones, onion, carrot tops, celery, white pepper, and a pinch of sugar – simmer for 1 hour and strain after cooking).

Divide the fish into small batches and mix in a food processor. Chop the fish, onions, and carrots. Transfer the mixture to an electric mixer. Add the eggs, salt, pepper, matzo meal, and a little ice water and beat well.

Dip hands in cold water and shape fish into balls. Place the balls in lightly boiling fish stock and cook uncovered for about 1 hour.

Or, for fish patties, shape the raw mixture into patties. Coat in matzo meal and fry in oil until light brown on each side, about 1 to 2 minutes per side. Finish by baking patties in a 350° oven for about 30 minutes.

TIPS & TRICKS:

- After mixing all the fish ingredients, taste a small portion raw and adjust seasonings.
- The balls don't freeze well, but the patties do. Freeze after frying, then thaw before baking.

MAMA'S GEFILTE FISH

Mary Noble

"My mother, Shyfra Knobel, is a Holocaust survivor. She grew up in a traditional family in Lelov, a small town in Poland. She and her family were routed from their home on Rosh Hashanah in 1939. She was 16 years old at the time. She spent the war years in a Czenstochova concentration camp, working in a munitions factory under horrific conditions. She met my father, Nechemia Knobel, in a DP (displaced persons) camp in Germany. They married, and my brother was born in Frankfurt, Germany, my sister in Israel, and I was born in Toronto after they emigrated to Canada. My mother was, and still is, a great cook, always making everything from scratch, including gefilte fish, typically made from white fish and pike.

"I married, and my husband and I moved to Spokane in 1979. We were invited to Bert Diskin's home for lunch after Rosh Hashanah, and for the first time I experienced gefilte fish made with salmon. It tasted fine, but it just wasn't the gefilte fish I grew up with. My parents came to visit me in Spokane soon after that. We went to the grocery store, and my mother started pointing to items at the fish counter saying, 'I'll take a pound of that and that and that.' It turned out to be cod, sole, and red snapper. She proceeded to make her gefilte fish, sweet, light, and yummy. It took me a while to fine tune the recipe because she made it using a 'juice glass of this and a big spoonful of that.'
Now I make her gefilte fish for our Seders every year."

Makes 30 balls

Fish:
½ carrot or less, peeled and cut into 1-inch pieces
1 large onion
6 stalks celery, cut into 1-inch pieces
1 pound each fresh cod, sole, and snapper
6 eggs
½ cup sugar
1½ cups matzo meal
¼ cup oil
3 teaspoons salt
¼ teaspoon pepper

In a food processor, process the carrots until very finely chopped. Remove to a bowl large enough to hold all the fish. Repeat this process with the onion and celery, making sure there are no remaining big chunks.

Process the fish until finely ground. You may want to do this in batches.

Add the fish to the vegetables, blending well. Add the eggs, sugar, matzo meal, oil, salt, and pepper. Mix by hand until thoroughly blended. Refrigerate for several hours or overnight.

Stock:
1 medium onion, chopped
2 extra-large carrots, sliced diagonally into 1-inch slices
3 stalks celery, cut into 1-inch pieces
3 tablespoons sugar
1 teaspoon salt
Pinch of pepper

Fill a large stockpot half-full with water. Add the onion, carrot, celery, sugar, salt, and pepper. Bring to a boil and simmer for 1 hour.

Form the fish mixture into balls and drop 10 pieces at a time into the boiling stock. Return the stock to a boil in between each addition.

Cover and simmer for 2 hours. Cool the fish in the pot completely before removing it to a storage container. Place the carrots and some broth over the fish and refrigerate until ready to use. Serve each ball with a carrot slice.

JERRY CONE'S GEFILTE FISH

Jerry Cone

"When I was a student at the University of Washington, I tried to arrange my classes to be in my Aunt Bertha Mosler's kitchen every Friday shortly after noon. Every Friday of my Aunt's married life, she made gefilte fish for Sabbath dinner. The fragrance of those fish balls simmering on the stove almost 75 years ago still drifts in and out of my memory. I've tried many times to recreate that aroma. The mixture is made from two of the richest fish in the sea, high in oil, gently combined and poached for the shortest possible time in a bath of flavorful fish stock. We serve it at holiday dinners, with the traditional horseradish and at other times with a spicy salsa."

Makes 24 balls

Stock:
Fish heads, bones, and skin
2 carrots, peeled and cut in 1-inch pieces
2 stalks celery (with leafy tops), quartered
2 small onions, quartered
½ bunch parsley, very coarsely chopped
1 tablespoon kosher salt

Put the fish heads, bones, skin, carrots, celery, onions, parsley, salt, and enough water to cover in a large soup pot. Bring to a boil and simmer for 30 minutes. Strain and reserve the stock and carrots to use for garnish.

Fish:
1 large onion, halved
1½ pounds wild King salmon, boned, skinned, and cut into chunks
1½ pounds Black Cod, boned, skinned, and cut into chunks
3 eggs
2 teaspoons kosher salt
1 teaspoon lemon pepper
1 teaspoon Old Bay Seasoning
¼ teaspoon cayenne pepper
¼ to ½ cup matzo meal, as needed

Process ½ of the onion in a food processor until fine. Add ½ of the salmon and ½ of the black cod and finely process. Transfer to a large bowl. Repeat the process with the remaining onion and fish.

Add the eggs, salt, Old Bay, lemon pepper, and cayenne pepper to the fish mixture. Add the matzo meal sparingly to make a workable mixture. Mix thoroughly.

Dip hands in cold water so fish doesn't stick to your fingers. Shape handfuls of the fish into desired ball size (the fish will expand). Drop the balls into boiling fish stock. Cover and reduce heat to simmer. Cook for 20 to 30 minutes.

Remove fish balls to a dish, adding enough stock to keep the fish moist. Let the fish cool then cover and refrigerate. Serve garnished with the reserved carrot pieces.

SALMON PATTIES

Tina Lippman Kahn

Makes approximately 20 patties

4 6-ounce cans red salmon, drained, skin and large bones removed
¼ teaspoon white pepper
2 teaspoons kosher salt
1½ cups matzo meal
2 lemons, juiced
4 eggs, beaten
1 large sweet onion, puréed
½ cup parsley, chopped
2 large yellow onions, sliced
½ cup canola oil plus more if needed
Lemon wedges, as garnish

Mash the salmon in a large bowl. Add the pepper, salt, matzo meal, lemon juice, eggs, onions, and parsley. Form the mixture into patties that are 4 inches in diameter and no more than ¾ inch thick.

Working in batches, heat enough oil to generously cover the bottom of a large pan. Spread a layer of sliced onions on the bottom of the pan. Place salmon patties on top of the onions and fry over medium heat until cooked through and golden on both sides. Blot the patties and onions on paper towels and place the patties and onions in a 9x13-inch pan. Add more sliced onions with each batch of patties. Several pans can be used at the same time to make the job go faster. If you wish, you can keep the patties warm in a 180° oven until all the patties are done.

Serve the patties cold, at room temperature, or warm from the oven. Serve with a plate of lemon wedges to squeeze on top.

SALMON WITH DILLED MAYONNAISE

Frances Rogers

"I have been making my fresh salmon recipe for many, many years. It is particularly popular as a Northwest favorite; after all, what's better than fresh salmon on a sunny, summer evening? Occasionally, I'd try to prepare a different menu to entertain my mahjongg and bridge club. They would quickly protest saying, 'You're going to make the fish, aren't you?' As time went on, it became apparent that mayonnaise, a key ingredient for this recipe, was becoming less popular. My children convinced me to try to make the fish with a slightly healthier twist: low fat mayo. It worked. They loved it, and the salmon dish lives on."

Serves 12 to 15

6 pounds fresh salmon, filleted and sliced in half lengthwise
½ teaspoon salt
½ teaspoon pepper
½ cup onion flakes
1 teaspoon dried dill weed
½ to ¾ cup mayonnaise, regular or low fat
¼ teaspoon onion salt
½ lemon, juiced
¼ teaspoon paprika
½ cup Parmesan cheese, grated (optional)

The night before, prepare a rimmed baking sheet by double lining it with foil. Spray the foil with nonstick spray. Place the salmon skin-side down on the foil and season it with the salt, pepper, onion flakes, and dill weed. Refrigerate.

When ready to bake, preheat the oven to 450°.

Bring the salmon to room temperature before cooking. Mix the mayonnaise, onion salt, lemon juice, paprika, and Parmesan cheese, if desired. Spread this mixture on top of the salmon. Bake the fish for 20 minutes. Check for doneness and continue cooking if necessary.

STEAMED SALMON

Sheila Sternberg

Serves 6 to 8

6 red lettuce leaves
1 3½-pound salmon filet
Kosher salt
12 round slices, fresh ginger, peeled plus 3 1-inch pieces, peeled
6 green onions, julienned, plus some cut at an angle, as a garnish
½ cup regular or light soy sauce
1 cup peanut oil (less if preferred)

Line the top basket of a steamer with the lettuce. Season the salmon filets with the salt and place them on the lettuce. Cover the filets with the ginger slices and green onions. Fill the bottom of the steamer with water and add the 3 pieces of ginger. Steam the salmon, covered, for about 18 minutes, until it flakes and is not red inside.

Place the salmon on a serving platter. Top with the remaining green onions. Pour the soy sauce over the salmon. Heat the peanut oil to a very hot temperature, pour it over the salmon, and serve. Garnish with a few more green onions.

GRILLED SALMON WITH BROWN SUGAR MUSTARD GLAZE

Sheila Sternberg

"I taught a salmon cooking class in 2004 for over 50 people. Among the attendees was the late great food writer, Eileen Mintz. Soon after this class, two of my recipes appeared in her Mercer Island Reporter *column, along with noted chefs from Salty's, Kasper Donier, and cookbook writer Rex Braiden-Johnson. I created the Grilled Salmon with Brown Sugar Mustard Glaze and recreated the steamed salmon recipe made in Chinese restaurants. I heard that there was a run on bamboo steamers bought right after this class. These recipes were served at the class with steamed white rice and bok choy."*

Makes 3 servings

¼ cup brown sugar
1 tablespoon honey
2 tablespoons butter
2 tablespoons Dijon mustard
1 tablespoon soy sauce
1 tablespoon olive oil
2 teaspoons fresh ginger, peeled and chopped
1 pound salmon

In a small saucepan over medium heat, melt the brown sugar, honey, and butter. Remove from the heat and add the mustard, soy sauce, olive oil, and ginger and blend well.

Place the salmon on a piece of heavy duty aluminum foil. Spread the glaze over the salmon. Barbecue over medium-high heat for about 12 minutes, basting often.

SALMON WITH SUN-DRIED TOMATOES

Loretta Kuznetz

"Over the years, I have passed this great recipe on to many people. It is perfect for the Pacific Northwest."

Serves 6 to 9

5 large cloves garlic, minced
3 tablespoons parsley, finely chopped
4 sun-dried tomatoes, packed in oil and finely chopped
1 teaspoon salt
¼ cup olive oil
1 2- to 3-pound salmon fillet

Combine the garlic, parsley, sun-dried tomatoes, salt, and oil in a jar. Let this mixture stand overnight in the refrigerator.

Place the salmon, skin side down, on a large piece of greased foil. Place the fish over low heat on the barbecue. Close the lid and cook for 10 minutes.

With a sharp knife cut 2 lengthwise slits in the fillet, dividing the surface of the fish in thirds. Cut to the skin, but not through it.

Spread the garlic mixture over all of the fillet and into the slits. Close the lid and increase the temperature to medium. Cook for an additional 15 minutes, until the fish flakes easily with a fork.

HALIBUT WITH HEAVENLY TOPPING

Marleen Alhadeff

"We first tried this recipe at Yes Bay Lodge, Alaska, where we fished for our dinner and planned our wedding over three decades ago. It has been a family favorite for all these years."

Serves 6

1 2-pound halibut fillet
2 tablespoons lemon juice
½ cup Parmesan cheese, grated
4 tablespoons butter, softened
3 tablespoons mayonnaise
3 tablespoons green onion, chopped
1 teaspoon Dijon mustard
¼ teaspoon salt
Dash of Tabasco sauce

Rinse and pat dry the fish. Place the fish in a single layer in a well-greased shallow baking dish. Brush with the lemon juice. Broil 4 inches from heat for 6 to 8 minutes.

Mix the Parmesan cheese, butter, mayonnaise, green onion, Dijon mustard, salt, and Tabasco sauce in a bowl and spread the cheese mixture on the fish.

Broil 2 to 3 minutes or until done.

Biscochos to Biscotti, Brownies to Burmuelos

Scent and memory are closely linked, and a particular smell has the ability to catapult us back to childhood and trigger the memories of people and places from our young worlds where we first absorbed it. It's no wonder, then, that this chapter – whose pages practically emit aromas of vanilla and sugar – churns up so much nostalgia.

An overwhelming number of these recipes conjure the legacies of grandmothers and mothers. Laurie Kever recalls her grandmother's unique preparations that rubbed off on her, like scraping the last bit of egg out of the egg shell, which years later she catches herself doing.

Other stories telescope into the early days of marriage: Joan Garden remembers the woman who mentored her as a young bride on how to make rugelah; Jane Isenberg revisits the cookbook her mother gave her as a newlywed and the brownie recipe she has passed down to her own daughter and granddaughter. And of course, the chain would not be complete without the stories of mothers baking with their daughters. Elise Topp remembers her freezer packed with shoeboxes of cookies, to be taken out by her daughters on the day of a party and artfully arranged on platters.

And then there are the recipes themselves: Traditional Sephardic round, crispy biscochos, served with sisterly rivalry; sutlach; and marzipan, whose almond base represents life and health. From Europe come those Jewish bakery stand-bys, cinnamon-rolled rugelah, bulging hamantashen, and crunchy mandelbreit/kamishbrot. No Washington State cookbook would be complete without a recipe for matzo roca, a Passover variation on Almond Roca®; neither would any be worthy of publishing without a good chocolate chip cookie. In this case, our submitters spent decades toiling over gooey spoons and bowls-in-need-of-licking to come up with the ultimate cookie experience. Aren't you glad they took the work out of it for you?

Most of these recipes don't stand out as "foodie." Instead they honor the conventional cooking wisdom of the mavens who inherited or created them. But leave it to one of our two male contributors to this chapter to throw a wrench into how we understand mavens and foodies. Dan Mintz shares Eileen Mintz's prize-winning chocolate rugelah, describing her as "a foodie long before anyone ever coined the term."

TIDBIT:
Rugelah, a Yiddish word probably derived from "spiral" or "twist," is native to Russia, Poland, and Ukraine. Its German equivalent is schneken, meaning "snail." Though they may be indecipherable now, they undergo different ways of cutting and rolling. Not to mention that American bakers constantly update the old-world recipe with new fillings.

BISCOCHOS TO BISCOTTI, BROWNIES TO BURMUELOS

BISCOCHOS

Esther Maimon

"My mother's, Sema Calvo, biscochos were legendary. She not only always had them in her home to offer to family and guests, but frequently gave them away to special people in her life, including her doctors. She was a welcome sight with her green MJB® coffee can in hand filled with her delicious biscochos. This recipe is a slight variation of my mother's and came from her sister, my aunt Betty Alhadeff. The two sisters were very competitive when it came to their baking and would frequently attempt to get an answer to the question, 'Whose biscochos are better?' We were all smart enough to know better than to answer that question."

Makes about 50 cookies

3 eggs, well beaten
Scant 3/4 cup sugar
3/8 cup oil
3 cups flour
1 heaping teaspoon baking powder

Preheat the oven to 350°. Mix the eggs, sugar, and oil well, slowly adding the flour and baking powder, which have been mixed together. Dough is ready when it cleans the side of the bowl and is no longer sticky.

Lightly dust a cutting board. Take a small amount of dough and roll into a log about the diameter of a quarter. Cut the log into pieces about 1 inch in length (to keep the biscochos smaller). Cover the remaining dough in the bowl to keep it from drying out.

Take one of the pieces and roll it into a log about 5 to 6 inches long. (If the dough is too soft, add a small amount of flour.) Flatten the log using your index and middle fingers, then fold the flattened log in half widthwise. Connect the two ends to form a circle and cut slits about 3/4 the way through the dough, about 1/3-inch apart.

1 egg, well beaten
1/8 teaspoon sugar
1 cup unbleached sesame seeds

Beat the egg and sugar together. Brush the tops of formed biscochos with egg mixture, and turn egg side down into plate of sesame seeds.

TIPS & TRICKS:

- Jeannie Alhadeff uses 1 teaspoon vanilla and ½ cup toasted sesame seeds (for the topping) in her biscocho recipe, which comes from her mother, Rosie Newhouse.
- You can make them any size and thickness you prefer.
- Do not use too much flour, or the biscochos will be too hard.
- When you cut each end diagonally, the circle fits together better.

Place the biscochos on a lightly floured, rimmed baking sheet (keeps the seeds in), leaving 1 inch between cookies.

Bake until lightly browned, about 15 to 20 minutes. Remove from pan and cool. Lower heat to 250°. Place cooled biscochos standing up on their side in rows in the baking pan. Place the pan in the oven and turn the heat off. Allow cookies to toast for 3 to 4 hours.

Cool and place in an airtight container.

ALMOND, RASPBERRY, AND DARK CHOCOLATE BISCOTTI

Karen Hudesman

"My daughters and I love to read cooking magazines together. We came across this very special biscotti recipe many years ago, and we decided to make it together. As we always do, we substituted some of the nuts, fruits, and chocolates to suit our taste and creativity. Every time I make this tasty cookie, I am not only reminded of the joys of my girls, but of my joy to try new things and my passion for baking."

Makes about 3 dozen cookies

3 cups all-purpose flour
2 teaspoons baking powder
½ teaspoon salt
1 cup sugar
3 large eggs
2 tablespoons canola oil
2½ teaspoons almond extract
¾ cup raw almonds, chopped
1 cup dried raspberries or dried strawberries, chopped (about 5 ounces)
1 pound plus ½ cup high-quality semisweet or bittersweet chocolate, chopped

Preheat the oven to 350°. Line a large baking sheet with parchment paper.

Whisk the flour, baking powder, and salt in a medium bowl. In the large bowl of an electric mixer, beat the sugar, eggs, oil, and almond extract until well blended. Add the flour mixture and beat until smooth. Stir in the almonds, dried berries, and ½ cup of the chocolate.

Drop dough by heaping tablespoons in two 12-inch-long strips onto the prepared baking sheet, spacing strips 3 inches apart. Using wet fingertips, shape each strip into a 3-inch-wide log, pressing evenly (the logs may be slightly lumpy).

Bake the logs for about 30 minutes, until lightly browned and almost firm to the touch. Cool the logs on the baking sheet for 30 minutes. Reduce the oven temperature to 325°.

Carefully transfer the logs to a cutting board. Line the same baking sheet with new parchment paper. Cut each log crosswise into generous ½-inch-thick slices. Stand the slices upright, spaced about ¼ inch apart, on the prepared baking sheet. Bake for about 20 minutes, until the biscotti are a pale, golden color. Cool completely on the baking sheet. They may be soft but will firm as they cool.

Put the remaining pound of chocolate in a microwave-safe glass bowl. Microwave on medium power in 30-second intervals, stirring well after each increment, until the chocolate is soft to the touch, about 2 minutes in total. Do not overheat or the chocolate will burn. Stir until the chocolate is smooth.

Line another large baking sheet with parchment paper. Dip one end or one side of each biscotti into the chocolate, then place it on the baking sheet. Chill the biscotti about 30 minutes, until the chocolate is set.

TIPS & TRICKS:

- The original recipe calls for pistachios and white chocolate, but I don't like white chocolate, and I prefer almonds to pistachios. Any dried berry is good, too.
- Biscotti can be made ahead. Arrange them in a single layer in an airtight container and store chilled up to 5 days or frozen up to 2 weeks.

KAMISHBROT

Marjorie Danz

"This is a recipe given to me by my mother, Eleanor Cohen. It is in her handwriting, but she got it from either her mother, Sadie Esfeld, or one of her four aunts. Mom used to make these by the pan full, and the aroma of cinnamon-sugar would fill the house. When I bake them now, the same aroma triggers the memory of having them baked as a child."

Makes 3 dozen cookies

3 eggs
1¼ cups sugar, divided
1 cup oil
1 teaspoon baking powder
1 teaspoon vanilla
Pinch of salt
1 cup almonds, sliced
3 cups flour, sifted
1 teaspoon cinnamon

Preheat the oven to 350°.

Beat the eggs, add 1 cup of the sugar, oil, baking powder, salt, and vanilla. Beat well with a wooden spoon. Fold in the nuts and enough flour to make a very stiff dough.

Shape into three long rolls on a baking sheet lined with parchment paper. Bake for 20 minutes, making sure not to brown. Remove the cookies from the oven and let cool for 15 minutes, until you can slice through without breaking.

Mix the remaining ¼ cup of sugar with the cinnamon and sprinkle over the sliced cookies.

Lower the oven temperature to 250°. Stand the sliced pieces up on a baking sheet and let the kamishbrot bake for another 1 to 1½ hours. Store in airtight containers.

TIPS & TRICKS:

❖ These can be freshened in the oven.

SYLVIA SAFRON'S MANDELBREIT

Carol Gown

"My mom, Sylvia Safron, of blessed memory, lived in Flushing, New York, and in the 35 years that we've lived in Seattle, she visited us here at least 50 or 60 times. She loved to bake and cook for us when she visited, and she loved when people expressed pleasure over her cooking and baking. I find that I think of my mom most acutely and sweetly when I cook with her recipes. Then, the memories of her pleasure in providing good food for her family – one way she demonstrated love to her children and her grandchildren – are the strongest.

One of my mom's signature desserts was her mandelbreit. She wrapped it in waxed paper and then tin foil, and brought it with her on the plane when she visited Seattle. She also baked it when she was in Seattle. This year for Rosh Hashanah, I made a double recipe of my mom's mandelbreit. My Seattle friends and family all fondly remembered Bubi as we enjoyed it. I then brought some back with me to New York when I visited my sister and her family in Brooklyn at Sukkot. In the sukkah, we ate my mom's stuffed cabbage, which my sister made, and my mom's mandelbreit, which I made. My mom was very much present with us that night."

Makes 6 dozen cookies

Filling:
¼ cup sugar
1 teaspoon cinnamon
½ to 1 cup jam (strawberry, raspberry, whatever your preference)
¼ to ½ cup walnuts, chopped

Mix the sugar and cinnamon and set aside. Mix the jam and walnuts and set aside. (Note: Mix some jam and some chopped nuts to get a desired "nuttiness"; there is no right way to do this.)

Dough:
4 eggs
1 cup sugar
1 cup margarine
1 teaspoon vanilla
4 cups flour
Vegetable oil
2 teaspoons baking powder

Preheat the oven to 350°.

Thoroughly mix the eggs, sugar, margarine, and vanilla. Combine the flour and baking powder. Add to the egg mixture and mix well.

Using vegetable oil on your hands to handle the dough, divide the dough into 6 parts. Shape each part into a "roll" and flatten out on a baking sheet. Using a spoon, spread a filling – either or both cinnamon-sugar or jam and nuts – down the center of each flattened loaf. Experimentation is okay and works. Pull the two sides together and pinch closed. Sprinkle the top of loaves with the cinnamon-sugar mixture.

Bake for 25 minutes. Cool slightly and then, using a sharp knife, cut each loaf into ½-inch-wide slices. Put the pans back in the oven and bake an additional 10 minutes. Cool.

RUGELAH

Joan Garden

"When I was 23 and newly married, my husband and I moved from St. Louis to Syracuse. Sadly, I had left my beloved family behind in St. Louis. But I met a Jewish woman in my new neighborhood, also named Joan, who was older and a great deal wiser. She took me under her wing and performed a mitzvah by teaching me how to bake. One of the recipes was this one for rugelah from the Syracuse newspaper. Several months later, my grandmother, Josie, who had arrived in St. Louis from Prague at the turn of the century, came to visit us in Syracuse and was delighted when she tasted the rugelah, stating it reminded her of the delicious pastry she was taught to bake by her grandmother. It gave her warm feelings of the past for her family, and I have to say, it does the same for me."

Makes 3 dozen cookies

Dough:
1 cup butter, softened
1 egg, separated
⅔ cup sour cream
2 cups flour

Place butter in a food processor and pulse until smooth.

Combine the egg yolk and sour cream in a small bowl. Refrigerate the egg white for later use.

Add the flour and sour cream mixture alternately to the butter and pulse just until the dough comes together in a ball. Divide the dough into three equal parts and wrap each in waxed paper. Refrigerate for at least 3 hours.

Filling:
¾ cup ground pecans or walnuts
2 tablespoons plus 1 teaspoon cinnamon
1 cup sugar, divided

Combine the nuts and 2 tablespoons of the cinnamon and ¾ cup of the sugar in a bowl and set aside. In a separate small bowl, combine the remaining teaspoon of cinnamon with the remaining ¼ cup of sugar and set aside.

When ready to bake, preheat the oven to 400°. Grease or line a baking sheet with parchment paper.

On a heavily floured board, or between two sheets of floured wax paper, roll out one section at a time of the cold dough into a 12-inch round shape. Using a floured pizza cutter, cut the dough into 8 wedges. Sprinkle the dough with one-third of the nut filling. Roll the dough from the outer edge of the piece to the inner point, shaping into a crescent shape and tucking the points under. Place on the baking sheet.

Beat the egg white then brush it over the top of the rugelah. Sprinkle with the cinnamon-sugar mixture. Bake until nicely browned, about 12 to 15 minutes.

EILEEN MINTZ'S PRIZE-WINNING CHOCOLATE CHIP COFFEE RUGELAH

Dan Mintz

"*Eileen Mintz was a foodie long before anyone ever coined the term and a maven whose excellent recipes were shared in her food column in the* Mercer Island Reporter. *Among her most famous culinary accomplishments is this recipe for her award-winning chocolate chip coffee rugelah. But it was her big and easy smile and loving nature that always warmed the hearts of all who knew her.*"

Makes 50 to 60 cookies

Dough:
1 cup butter, room temperature
8 ounces cream cheese, room temperature
1 teaspoon vanilla
3 tablespoons chocolate topping or sauce
2 cups unbleached flour

In the bowl of an electric mixer, cream the butter, then add the cream cheese, vanilla, and chocolate. Add the flour and mix well.

Remove the dough from the bowl, form into five equal pieces, and flatten into disks. Wrap each piece in plastic and refrigerate for 6 hours or overnight.

Filling:
12 ounces bittersweet chocolate chips
7 teaspoons cinnamon, divided
¾ cup pecans, toasted and chopped
4 tablespoons instant coffee or espresso crystals
1 cup sugar, divided
4 tablespoons butter, melted and cooled
¼ cup canola oil, for brushing

Using a food processor, crush the chocolate chips. Then add 4 teaspoons of the cinnamon, pecans, coffee, ½ cup of the sugar, and butter and process into a paste. Set aside. In a separate small bowl, combine the remaining 3 teaspoons of the cinnamon with the remaining ½ cup of the sugar and set aside.

Preheat the oven to 350°. Line 2 baking sheets with parchment paper.

On a floured board, roll each dough disc into an 8-inch circle. Lightly brush each circle with oil. Sprinkle each circle with the cinnamon-sugar mixture and cut each circle into 12 wedges with a pizza cutter. Place 1 tablespoon of the filling at the wide edge of each of the wedges and roll up. Brush the top lightly with oil and sprinkle with more of the cinnamon-sugar mixture. Repeat until all the dough is used.

Bake for 15 to 20 minutes, until lightly browned. Cool on wire racks.

TIPS & TRICKS:

- To toast the pecans, place them on a baking sheet in a 325° oven and cook until lightly browned.
- Once cooled completely, the rugelah will freeze well in plastic freezer bags.

MY MOTHER'S CREAM CHEESE COOKIES

Joyce Dickhaut

"These cookies are a wonderful memory from my childhood. When I got home from school and saw a cube of butter and a block of cream cheese softening in a bowl on the kitchen counter, I knew it was just a matter of time before we would be enjoying these yummy cookies."

Makes 12 cookies

½ cup butter
1 3-ounce package cream cheese
1 cup flour
½ cup raspberry jam
Powdered sugar, for dusting

Preheat the oven to 400°. Line a baking sheet with parchment paper.

Let the butter and cream cheese sit at room temperature until they are soft enough to stir together. Cream the butter and cream cheese.

Blend in the flour and form the dough into a ball. If too soft, chill slightly then roll out on a floured board with a rolling pin until the dough is the thickness of a pie crust. Cut into 2-inch squares. Place a small dab of jam in the center of each square (a little jam goes a long way) and roll diagonally, pinching the ends together, and bend so they look like little crescent rolls.

Bake for 10 minutes, until just golden. Do not let them get brown. When they come out of the oven, dust the cookies with powdered sugar, cool, then serve.

TIPS & TRICKS:

- You can roll this dough in a circle, cut the wedges, place ½ teaspoon of jam on the wide edge, and roll from the wide edge to the inner point.

HAMANTASHEN WITH COTTAGE CHEESE PASTRY

Fred Maslan

"My mom, Florence Maslan, used to make these for Purim, and I remember them fondly. They are smaller than traditional Hamentashen so you can pop them into your mouth whole."

Makes 2 dozen cookies

1 cup butter, room temperature
1 cup low fat cottage cheese, room temperature
½ cup sugar
2½ cups flour
½ teaspoon salt
¾ cup jam of your choice

Preheat the oven to 350°. Line 2 baking sheets with parchment paper.

In a food processor, combine the butter, cottage cheese, and sugar until well blended. Add the flour and salt and mix just until a ball forms. Wrap the dough in plastic and refrigerate at least 1 hour.

Roll out the dough as you would a pie crust, about ⅛-inch-thick. With a cookie cutter, cut into 2-inch rounds. Put the jam of your choice in the center and form into hamentashen. Seal and bake for 12 to 15 minutes, until lightly browned.

HAMANTASHEN

Pip and Miriam Meyerson

"My mother, who lives in Vancouver, BC, would try to get the cookie dough as thin as possible, by rolling each circle after cutting them out. She was a fantastic baker. We once catered a wedding and instead of a wedding cake, the family wanted traditional Jewish baking. She came to Seattle, and we spent the entire day in the kitchen, creating an assortment of desserts that were the highlight of the wedding."

Makes 2 to 3 dozen cookies

Filling:
½ pound pitted prunes
½ cup raisins
½ cup walnuts or almonds, very finely chopped
1 lemon, juiced and rind grated
½ cup sugar

Soak the prunes and raisins in water to cover overnight. Drain and discard the liquid. Combine the prunes, raisins, nuts, lemon juice, and rind in a food processor and blend.

Dough:
3 eggs plus 1 egg, for brushing
½ cup sugar
½ cup oil
1 teaspoon vanilla
1 orange, juiced and rind grated
2½ to 3 cups of flour
2 teaspoon baking powder
¼ teaspoon salt

Preheat the oven to 350°.

Mix 3 of the eggs, sugar, oil, vanilla, orange juice, and rind together in a large bowl. Sift the flour, baking powder, and salt together before adding to the wet ingredients, using only enough flour to handle.

Flour a work board and roll the dough to ¼-inch thickness. Use a 2-inch or larger glass to cut circles. Spoon 1 teaspoon of the filling into the middle of each circle and fold into triangle by pinching the dough together, top half first, then bringing bottom flap up. Pinch the corners together tightly or they will open during baking.

Beat the remaining egg and brush the top of each hamentashen. Bake in the upper third of oven for 25 minutes, until golden brown.

BUBBA SHULMAN'S HAMANTASHEN

Julie Katz

"My grandmother, Hanna Kurinetsky Shulman, was born in Russia in 1898. Her father was burned alive in a synagogue with countless other Jewish men when she was 28 days old. She lived through the Russian Revolution and two world wars, going into hiding in Russian swamps to flee the Nazis, living for years on cranberries and whatever else they could find to eat. Bubba and her family made their way to Shlachtansee, a displaced persons camp in Berlin in 1945, and sailed for the U.S. in 1947.

"When she arrived in Seattle, where her brothers-in-law lived, she went to work in a pickle factory, ever grateful to be in this great country. Bubba was a second mother to me and my two sisters, always loving, listening to, and believing in us. She and Zaydeh never learned to drive, but would take us downtown on the bus to the bank, out to lunch, to the Pike Place Market for ice cream. Every weekend, we spent the night at their house, walking to synagogue with them on Saturdays and enjoying unlimited amounts of homemade blintzes, bagels, challah, taiglach, milchikeh (yeast coffee cake), mandelbreit, chicken soup, borscht, and lemon meringue pie. They grew their own raspberries, roses, peonies, tomatoes, nasturtiums, and garlic, and canned their own peaches and cherries. Bubba made her own loktion (pasta) and blackberry wine. She would tell us stories of her survival during the day, and sing Yiddish, Russian, and White Russian folk songs to us before bed at night. When we earned our drivers' licenses as teenagers, we were allowed to drive to certain destinations only, and of course, Bubba and Zaydeh's house was on the short list.

"One of her recipes that I make each year is Bubba's Hamantashen. The dough is foolproof, and I fill it with all kinds of fillings, not just the traditional ones. Enjoy!"

Makes about 3 dozen cookies

Filling:
½ pound yellow raisins
1 pound prunes, pitted
½ pound dates, pitted
½ cup walnuts, ground
½ lemon, including rind
½ orange, including rind
1 tablespoon red wine
¼ cup raspberry jam
Honey and/or sugar, to taste

Soak the raisins and prunes in water or orange juice for 30 to 40 minutes, until they are plump and soft. Drain and discard the liquid.

Grind the raisins, prunes, dates, nuts, lemon, and the orange until the pieces are about the size of a pea – do not grind it until it is smooth. Add the wine, jam, and honey or sugar (if desired) at the end to achieve the proper taste and texture.

Dough:
¼ cup butter (shortening, if making pareve)
¼ cup oil
1 cup sugar
1 egg
2½ cups flour
2 teaspoons baking powder
¼ cup orange juice

Preheat the oven to 375°.

Cream the butter, oil, sugar, and egg. Combine the flour and baking powder in a separate bowl. Gradually add the flour to the butter mixture, alternating with the orange juice. Roll the dough out to ¼-inch thickness, adding more flour if the dough doesn't roll easily. Cut the dough into circles about 3-inches in diameter.

Fill the dough circles with a scant tablespoon of fruit filling and fold the sides inwards to form a triangle, pinching the edges to seal. Bake for 10 to 15 minutes.

TIPS & TRICKS:

- The recipe makes three times the amount of filling needed for the amount of dough so adjust accordingly.

MINT MERINGUES

Sherry Benaroya

"This has been my all-time favorite cookie since I was a little girl. In fact, I think it's the favorite of our entire extended family! They are nice and crisp on the outside and soft on the inside. The recipe, which is from my mother, Mary Berns, is great for Passover (using the appropriate chocolate), but I make it all year long."

Makes 2 dozen cookies

2 egg whites, beaten
1/8 teaspoon cream of tartar
3/4 cup ultra-fine sugar
1/2 teaspoon vanilla
Green food coloring
6 ounces minted chocolate chips (or substitute a mint chocolate bar, chopped)

Preheat the oven to 275°.

Beat the egg whites in an electric mixer on medium speed for a minute or two until the whites are thick and foamy, but not yet forming soft peaks. Add the cream of tartar, then 2 tablespoons of the sugar and beat well, increasing the speed from medium-high to high as you continue. Keep adding the sugar, 2 tablespoons at a time, beating well after each addition, until mixture is very thick and glossy and forms stiff peaks (this will take about 10 minutes).

Add the vanilla and the green food coloring to the desired shade. Gently fold in the chocolate chips.

Using a tablespoon, form into mounds (with or without peaks) on an ungreased baking sheet. Bake for 20 minutes, until firm.

TIPS & TRICKS:

- Use fresh egg whites that are at room temperature (cold whites tend to reduce the volume).
- Do not let even a drop of yolk get into the egg whites.
- I prefer using ultra-fine sugar because it dissolves more quickly than regular granulated sugar.

GRANDMA LIL'S SESAME COOKIES

Diane Cohn and Laurie Kever

"Grandma Lil, Elizabeth Cohn, was Jerry Cohn's mother. She was the *baker of the times. She baked for the servicemen during the war and delivered her baked goods.*

"Her granddaughter, Laurie Kever, tells this story: I learned to make these with my Grandma Lil when I was in college. I don't cook, so it was ironic that I would be the one to learn many of her baking recipes. While she was mixing the ingredients, she would do odd things (at least to me) such as scraping the inside of the egg shell to make sure she got every last drop of egg. I actually found myself doing that when I made cookies last night! It made me think of her and smile. This is my favorite of all of her cookie recipes – and she had a lot!"

Makes about 5 dozen cookies

1 egg
1 cup margarine or butter, softened
1 cup sugar
2 cups flour, sifted
½ teaspoon baking soda
½ teaspoon salt
1 teaspoon vanilla
1 to 2 cups sesame seeds

Blend the egg, margarine or butter, sugar, flour, baking soda, salt, and vanilla together in a large bowl. Cover and store in the refrigerator overnight or in the freezer for a few hours.

When ready to bake, preheat the oven to 350°.

Form the cookie dough into small balls and roll them in the sesame seeds until they are well coated. Put the cookies on a baking sheet and bake until they are brown, about 10 minutes or so.

"My grandmother (Nana), Minnie Allen Sherman, came with her family from Akkerman, Russia, to Portland, Oregon, at age 21, and spent the rest of her life there. In Russia, her father owned a bakery, and they also had servants. She didn't grow up baking, although as an adult, she did become a wonderful cook. She and my grandfather had a few small businesses over time, including a grocery store, and she delighted in discovering new fruits and vegetables. I remember her excitement when she was introduced to 'star fruit.' She passed along this ethic, and to this day in our family we call each other if we come across a new kind of fruit. Nana was a wonderful cook, and her meals were also healthy. She had many wonderful cookie recipes and baked a variety each week for the cookie trays served at the Friday night onegs at Congregation Neveh Shalom. In our family we especially remember her sesame cookies. She always had them on hand, kept in a black cloisonné-patterned tin canister, and ready for drop-in guests. They are not too big and not too rich, so you could eat a few of them and it was still a light dessert."

~ Carolyn Cohen

MOMMY'S BEST OATMEAL CHOCOLATE CHIP COOKIES

Lian Caspi

"These are cookies my mom baked all through my childhood. I make them even now as I am in college. They remind me of home. These are best with a glass of milk!"

Makes 2 dozen cookies

1 cup butter, room temperature
½ cup brown sugar
½ cup sugar
2 eggs
1 teaspoon vanilla
2 cups flour (1 cup can be whole wheat flour, if desired)
2 cups quick-cooking oatmeal
1 teaspoon baking powder
½ teaspoon baking soda
¼ cup milk
1 cup walnuts or pecans, chopped
1 to 2 cups semisweet chips

Preheat the oven to 350°. Grease 2 baking sheets.

Cream the butter, brown sugar, and sugar in a large bowl until fluffy. Add the eggs and vanilla and mix well.

In another bowl, mix the flour, oatmeal, baking powder, and baking soda. Alternately, add the dry ingredients and the milk to the sugar and butter mixture. Add the nuts and chocolate chips.

Drop by tablespoons onto the baking sheet 1-inch apart and bake for 15 minutes, until brown. Cool on wire racks.

THREE CHIP COOKIES

Lesley Masin Grosvenor

"Throughout my entire life – really – my mom, Cindy, has made it her mission to bake the perfect chocolate chip cookie – a cookie that is crispy on the outside and chewy on the inside, doesn't flatten out when baking, is loaded with chocolate chips, and is about 3 inches in diameter. So you can imagine the possibilities, not to mention pounds gained, to find the perfect cookie. Nestle's Tollhouse cookies used to be her standby, but this is the one she and I have been making lately (or at least until we find the next best)."

Makes about 30 cookies

1¼ cups all-purpose flour
1 teaspoon baking soda
½ teaspoon salt
½ cup unsalted butter, room temperature
½ cup golden brown sugar, firmly packed
6 tablespoons sugar
1 large egg
1 teaspoon vanilla
1 cup bittersweet chocolate chips
1 cup white chocolate chip
1 cup milk chocolate chips

Preheat the oven to 350°. Line 2 rimless baking sheets with parchment paper.

In a bowl, sift together the flour, baking soda, and salt. Set aside.

In an electric mixer fitted with the paddle attachment, combine the butter, brown sugar, and sugar. Beat on medium speed until smooth. Add the egg and vanilla and beat on low speed until well blended. Slowly add the dry ingredients and beat on low speed, just until incorporated. Add the bittersweet, white, and milk chocolate chips and mix again on low speed until the chips are incorporated.

Drop the dough by heaping tablespoons onto the prepared baking sheets, spacing the cookies about 2 inches apart. Bake the cookies, one sheet in the oven at a time, until they are an even golden brown, about 10 to 13 minutes. Let the cookies cool on the baking sheets for 5 minutes, then transfer them to wire racks to cool completely. Store in an airtight container at room temperature for up to 3 days or frozen in freezer bags.

TIPS & TRICKS:

- If you prefer, this can also be made in a 10x15-inch glass dish and cut into bars. For bars, spoon the entire mixture into a lightly buttered 10x15-inch glass dish. Bake at 350° for about 30 minutes, until brown all over and a toothpick inserted into the middle comes out clean.

DUTCH BUTTER COOKIES

Janet Gray

"My mom's, Arva Gray, greatest legacy was her family. She and my dad, Bernard, presided over the dining room table, which was always full of family, dear friends, and fabulous food. Mom's secret ingredient was love, and she heavily seasoned each dish with it. The cookie jar was constantly filled with Dutch Butter Cookies, a 'secret' recipe handed down from Aunt Freda Gray."

Makes 2 to 3 dozen cookies

1 cup butter
1 cup sugar
1 egg yolk (or 1 ounce egg beaters)
1½ cups filberts, toasted and chopped
½ cup poppy seeds
1 teaspoon vanilla
1¾ cups flour
½ teaspoon cinnamon
¼ teaspoon ginger
¼ teaspoon salt

Preheat the oven to 325°.

Cream the butter and sugar, then add the egg yolk. Stir in the filberts, poppy seeds, and vanilla. Gradually add the flour, cinnamon, ginger, and salt to make a firm, but sticky dough. Form five 1½ inch balls, wrap in wax paper, and chill for 4 hours.

Cut each dough ball into ¼-inch-thick slices and bake on ungreased baking sheets for 15 to 20 minutes, until light brown.

CHOCOLATE FROSTING COOKIES

Deanne Seinfeld Rubinstein

"This is a favorite recipe of my mother, Sylvia Seinfeld, who lived in Tacoma for 67 years. Sylvia loved storing Chocolate Frosting Cookies in her basement chest freezer so they would always be available when any of her grandchildren came to visit. They were never disappointed. In fact, now each of my 5 grandchildren loves baking this family favorite with me."

Makes 2 dozen cookies

1 cup margarine or butter, softened
1 cup brown sugar
1 egg, beaten
2 cups unbleached all-purpose flour, sifted
2 teaspoons vanilla
12 ounces semisweet chocolate chips

Preheat the oven to 350°.

In an electric mixer fitted with the paddle attachment, mix the butter, brown sugar, and egg. Gradually blend in the flour and then add the vanilla. Press the dough into a 9x13-inch pan using the back of a wet spoon. Bake for 12 to 15 minutes, until light brown. Turn off the oven.

Remove the pan from the oven and spread the chocolate chips evenly over the pan. Put the pan back in the oven for a couple of minutes, until the chocolate is spreadable. Cool on a rack until the chocolate hardens.

TIPS & TRICKS:

- Make small lines vertically and horizontally in the chocolate so when the cookies are cool they can be easily removed.
- You can use whole wheat flour.
- Shake sprinkles on top if you want to make them fancier.
- Refrigerate for quick cooling.

PEANUT BUTTER ADDICTION BARS

Jackie Goldfarb

"These cookies are my son Steven's favorite cookies. He always asked for them as a child and still has me make them today."

Makes 24 to 30 bars

1 cup sugar
1 cup corn syrup
1½ cups peanut butter
6 cups Special K® cereal
12 ounces chocolate chips
12 ounces butterscotch chips

Grease a 9x13x2-inch baking dish.

In a medium pot over low heat, mix the sugar, corn syrup, and peanut butter together until melted. Add the cereal, 1 cup at a time, and mix until combined. Press the cereal mixture into the baking dish.

In a separate bowl, melt the chocolate and butterscotch chips together. Pour the chocolate mixture on top of the cereal mixture. Cool. When the mixture hardens, cut into squares.

O'HENRY BARS
Gladys Rubinstein

Makes 24 to 30 bars

1 cup dark corn syrup
1 cup sugar
1⅓ cups peanut butter
5 cups corn flakes, coarsely crushed
6 ounces chocolate chips
6 ounces butterscotch chips

Grease a 9x13x2-inch baking dish.

Bring the corn syrup and sugar to a rolling boil. Remove from heat. Add the peanut butter and mix well.

Place the corn flakes in the baking dish and pour the peanut butter mixture over the cereal. Press to flatten.

Melt the chocolate and butterscotch chips together in a double boiler and pour over the cornflake mixture. Cool and cut into squares.

MILDRED LEVIN'S BROWNIES

Jane Isenberg

"In 2003, when my husband and I left the East Coast and moved to Issaquah, we brought along my stash of Jewish cookbooks. Included was a dog-eared and stained copy of Dining Out at Home *published by the Passaic (New Jersey) Section of the National Council of Jewish Women. My mother gifted me this book when I was a newlywed. Almost half a century later, my daughter, Rachel Stoner, and I still use it. Rachel's young daughter, Jordan, uses it too. Not surprisingly, one of Jordan's favorite recipes is for brownies. Mildred Levin, a friend of my mother's, contributed it. My mom used to send me these brownies when I was in college, and I sent them to Rachel when she went to college, and in time, God willing, we'll both send them to Jordan."*

Makes 24 to 36 brownies

4 ounces bittersweet chocolate
½ pound butter
4 eggs
2 cups sugar
1 cup flour, sifted
1 teaspoon vanilla
1 cup walnuts, chopped

Preheat the oven to 350°. Grease and flour an 8x11-inch pan.

Melt chocolate and butter in a double boiler. Cool.

Beat 1 egg well and gradually add the sugar. Add the other 3 eggs, one at a time, and combine with the chocolate mixture. Add the flour and mix until just blended. Add the vanilla and fold in the walnuts. Pour into the prepared pan and bake for 25 to 30 minutes. Cool on a rack.

TIPS & TRICKS:

❖ For really moist brownies, cover the pan of brownies while still warm and place in the refrigerator to chill for several hours. Cut into squares or bars when ready to serve.

SLICED ALMOND BARS

Elise Topp

"I grew up in Seattle, on Capitol Hill, very close to Volunteer Park. It was a lovely home with a substantial kitchen. And, while I would like to say that it was in that kitchen that my interest in cooking began, I must admit that is not the case. The reason for that interesting scenario was that my three sisters, brother, and I were not allowed in the kitchen. My parents employed a cook named Dora, who always wore a stiff white apron and a chef's hat, and had little tolerance for children underfoot.

"My mother, Rebecca Betty Shafer, would go into the kitchen every morning to plan the day's meals, and Dora would go off to the market and pick up the necessary ingredients. I fondly remember Dora's juicy roasted chicken and famous lemon meringue pie.

"When Bill Topp, an Air Force surgeon at the time, came into the family, he was allowed to take over the carving responsibilities from my father, Julius, who was happy to relinquish carving to a doctor who 'really knew what he was doing.' When Bill and I married in 1946, I knew it was time to learn about cooking, so I enrolled in a cooking class at Broadway High School. Slowly, but surely, and by trial and error, I learned to cook from my mother-in-law, Goldie Topolovitz, my sisters-in-law, Minnie Cohn and Esther Schwartz, and from the many, many cookbooks that became my constant inspiration. I would clip recipes from newspapers and magazines and I treasured the recipes I got from Minnie and Esther.

"As time went on, Bill and I established our own traditions. Every Friday night, our family would say the blessings while lighting the candles, breaking the bread, drinking sweet Manischewitz wine, and enjoying a meal of beef or chicken along with the new recipe du jour. I was always trying something new, and my family members were willing testers. I especially liked trying different cookie recipes. I loved to bake and would bake and freeze cookies for any big or small family occasion. Our freezer was always full of shoeboxes and shirt boxes filled with cookies. We entertained quite a lot and on the day of a party, my daughters and I would arrange dozens and dozens of cookies on platter after platter to serve for dessert, making sure the presentation of the cookies was as appealing as their sweet taste. My daughters and I still bake many of these recipes today."

Makes 24 bars

Crust:
½ cup butter
1¼ cups flour
¼ cup sugar
1 egg yolk, beaten
½ teaspoon vanilla

In a large bowl, cut the butter into the flour and sugar until coarse crumbs. Stir in the egg yolk and vanilla. Refrigerate the dough for at least 1 hour.

Topping:
3 tablespoons butter
2 tablespoons milk
½ cup sugar
1 tablespoon honey
1 cup sliced almonds

In a small pan, heat the butter and milk until the butter is melted. Add the sugar, honey, and almonds and stir well. Set aside.

When ready to bake, preheat the oven to 325°. Lightly butter a 9x9-inch pan.

Press the chilled dough into the pan, forming a bit of a rim. Bake for about 25 minutes, until just golden. Spread the filling over the warm pastry. Return the pan to the oven and bake another 20 to 30 minutes, until a rich brown.

When cooled, these can be cut into bars or larger squares. It also looks attractive as a whole torte served on a square plate.

PRUNE RIBBON COOKIE BARS

Jeanne Maimon

"I found this recipe in Good Housekeeping *magazine at least 25 years ago. We used to host a large open house each year on the night of Purim. The prune filling fit in with all the Purim goodies."*

Makes 27 bars

1 12-ounce package pitted prunes
1 cup water
¼ cup honey
¼ large lemon, unpeeled
2 cups flour
1½ cups light brown sugar, packed
¾ cup butter or margarine, softened
1 teaspoon baking powder
1 teaspoon vanilla
½ teaspoon salt
1 egg

Preheat the oven to 350°. Grease a 9x9-inch pan.

In a 2-quart saucepan over medium-high heat, heat the prunes and water until boiling. Reduce the heat to low, cover the pan, and simmer for 3 minutes. Drain the prunes well.

Blend the prunes, honey, and lemon in a food processor or blender at high speed until very smooth. Set aside.

Mix the flour, brown sugar, butter or margarine, baking powder, vanilla, salt, and egg in a large bowl of an electric mixer. Increase the speed to medium and beat until smooth, scraping the bowl occasionally. Divide the dough into three equal parts.

With greased fingers, press one-third of the dough into the bottom of the pan. With a spoon, carefully spread half of the prune mixture over the dough. Repeat and end with the dough.

Bake for 1 hour, until browned and the dough pulls away from the side of the pan.

Cool in the pan, on a wire rack. When ready to serve, cut into 3x1-inch bars. Store in a tightly covered container for up to two weeks or freeze.

MARZIPAN

Sharon Cordova Lott

*"Marzipan (*Masapan *in Ladino) is a sweet Sephardic confection traditionally served for important life cycle events like baby-namings, bar mitzvahs, and weddings. Marzipan represents good health and the celebration of life, as its key ingredient is almonds, which contain essential nutrients of life.* Con salute…*to your health!"*

Makes 45 to 50 pieces

2 cups slivered almonds, blanched
2 cups powdered sugar
2 egg whites from large eggs
Silver balls, for decoration

Line a baking sheet with parchment paper.

Grind the almonds in a food processor until very finely ground (like a fine powder). Add the powdered sugar and mix. Add the egg whites, one at a time, until the dough is smooth and forms a ball all by itself (usually about 1½ egg whites, plus a little).

Break the dough into large balls about the size of a small tennis ball. Form into long snakes about 1-inch in diameter. Use a sharp knife that has been dipped in very hot water and cut on the diagonal. Place one silver ball on top of each piece. Freeze on baking sheets and then place in containers for further freezing or transporting.

TIPS & TRICKS:

- Instead of almonds, use unsalted peanuts. Shape into small balls and top with a chocolate chip on each piece. Only marzipan can be in diagonal diamond shapes.

PASSOVER MATZO ROCA

Shelley Bensussen

Makes 40 to 50 pieces

5 sheets matzo
1 cup butter or margarine
1 cup brown sugar
1 12-ounce package semi-sweet chocolate chips
1 cup almonds or walnuts, chopped

Preheat the oven to 350°. Cover a baking sheet with aluminum foil, dull side up, and grease well. Place whole matzos on the foil in a single layer to cover the entire baking sheet, cutting extra pieces to fill any empty spaces.

Combine the butter and sugar in a saucepan over medium heat. Bring to a boil, stirring constantly, and boil for 4 to 5 minutes. Pour the caramel mixture evenly over the matzos, covering each sheet completely, and bake for 5 minutes.

Remove from the oven and immediately sprinkle with the chocolate chips; when the chips have softened, spread evenly with a knife over the caramel layer. Sprinkle the chopped nuts on the chocolate and freeze for 1 hour.

While still frozen, break the matzo roca into pieces and store in the freezer until ready to use.

TIPS & TRICKS:

- When making the caramel, be very careful, as the mixture becomes very hot.
- You can omit the chocolate and just sprinkle with the nuts.
- For a twist and added crunch, try using toasted nuts or using pecans.

CHOCOLATE, ALMOND, AND FARFEL BITES

Bobbie Stern

"One of my friends ran into my mom, Fern Meltzer, many, many years ago at the grocery store right before Passover. They traded stories, asking each other, 'How many people are you having?' 'What are you serving?' 'Do you have any great recipes I should try?' And according to my friend, my mom said, 'Yes. I have a recipe for you. Are you ready? It's very complicated.' My friend says that every year around Passover, she relives that moment in the grocery store with my mom as she easily makes this 'very complicated' recipe for chocolate almond farfel bites."

Makes 40 to 50 pieces

1⅓ cups matzo farfel
1⅓ cups slivered almonds
1 11½-ounce package chocolate chips (you can use semisweet, bittersweet, mint, or white)

Line a baking sheet with parchment paper.

Brown the matzo farfel and almonds separately in either a dry frying pan or on a rimmed baking sheet lined with foil in a 350° oven for about 15 minutes.

Melt the chocolate chips in a microwaveable bowl in 30-second increments, stirring between each interval, about 2 to 3 minutes total. Stir until smooth. Add the browned matzo farfel and almonds and mix until the farfel and almonds are completely covered in chocolate.

Drop by heaping teaspoons the baking sheet and refrigerate until the chocolate hardens.

LA DOUCE VIE FUDGE

Betsy R. Schneier, who learned it from Sarah Vyborny, her French teacher, and aunt of Janine Guttman Rosenbaum.

"At Roosevelt High School in the early 1970s, Madame Sarah Vyborny, my French teacher, had a formidable reputation as a tough teacher who was also a 'character.' Standing barely 5 feet tall, thanks to a bouffant hairstyle that never changed, she struck fear into the hearts of those who could not pick up the nuances of the dense literature she assigned us.

"We knew she wasn't born in France. I can vividly recall her Polish accent in both English and French. Only in later years did I learn more important facts about her life.

"She always kept a huge portrait of her niece, Janine, on her desk. Exactly why she was so fond of 'Jeh-nine' she never explained, but I discovered that Janine went to Israel and later married Rabbi Jay Rosenbaum, who became the Rabbi at Herzl-Ner Tamid Congregation. Janine, herself, is a master Jewish educator at Seattle Hebrew Academy.

"'Madame' never talked about children. We were her offspring, she always said. Occasionally she'd talk about a few relatives that she came over with from Europe, but as teens we never paid much attention. For those who struggled in her class, it took tremendous energy just to keep up with her assignments.

"Like most of the students who stayed with her through the years of high school, I adored her. The love was reciprocated, and at first I thought this was because I picked up foreign languages rather easily. Later on, though, she told me the truth – or at least bits of it. She was Jewish, and she knew I was too.

"Sarah Vyborny grew up in a large, high-achieving family in pre-war Poland. She became a judge, but when Hitler came to power, she went into the Warsaw Ghetto and then worked in forced labor camps. How she came to Seattle remained a mystery, until I met her sister Deborah. Thanks to Janine's family, I learned the whole story.

"Madame had been married, but her husband did not survive World War II. After the war, she met her 2nd husband Frank in Morocco, where she was working for the Joint Distribution Committee. Madame and Frank returned to Paris and married. Madame's sister Deborah and brother-in-law Victor Guttman also lived in Paris, where they gave birth to a daughter, Janine. Shortly afterwards, while Janine was still an infant, they were reunited with their brother, Albert, who had left Poland before the war, and was now an American G.I. Albert convinced the family to come to America rather than to Israel, as they had planned. Along with them came Madame's sister-in-law Bronislava (Bronka) and Bronka's 10-year-old son, Alex Sytman, who married Seattle native Lucy (Israel) Sytman and became one of Seattle's prominent cardiologists. Both her niece Janine and nephew Alex gave Madame tremendous naches.

"This fudge recipe figures into the tale because it served as the major fundraising vehicle for her brainchild at Roosevelt: La Douce Vie, *a literary magazine* en francais. *She implored many of us to submit our best work – poetry and prose – to be published in this journal. Although the principal admired her pluck, no funds were set aside for the French Department to publish anything in those days, so Madame decided to raise funds by selling fudge at intermission during Roosevelt's highly acclaimed dramatic presentations. When students wanted a break from Sartre, Dylan Thomas, and other 'serious' productions, they eagerly lined up for the fudge, and we always netted enough profits to publish another issue of* La Douce Vie.

"I make this fudge once a year. And, despite the fact that I rarely use ingredients like those she commanded us to incorporate, I do so anyway, in the spirit of Marcel Proust and his remembrances of things past."

1 13-ounce can evaporated milk
4½ cups sugar
1 cup margarine, melted
8 ounces marshmallows
24 ounces chocolate chips
2 cups walnuts or pecans, chopped
2 teaspoons vanilla
½ teaspoon salt

Grease a 9x13-inch pan.

In a small saucepan, bring the milk to a boil, then gradually add the sugar, stirring constantly, for approximately 10 minutes. Remove from heat and add the margarine, marshmallows, chocolate chips, nuts, vanilla, and salt. Stir vigorously for at least 5 minutes, before pouring into the pan. Cool completely before cutting.

CHOCOLATE MOUSSE

Emily Keeler Alhadeff

"When I became a vegetarian as a teenager in the mid-1990s, few options existed. Our local supermarket in small-town Connecticut carried a brand or two of veggie burgers, and I remember sitting down to holiday dinners with this dried-out, rubber, hockey puck of an excuse for my main dish.

"Over time, vegetarian cuisine reached gourmet heights. One summer, while working as a baker in a natural foods store, I discovered the art of vegan desserts. We used to sell this vegan mousse topped with chopped hazelnuts in little cups, and they flew off the shelves. Since then, it has become both my default and my specialty, loved even by the omnivorous people in my life who never trusted things like tofu. Tofu has the ability to impact people early on, but even the most traumatized will enjoy this (all the more so if you never tell them it's tofu!). It's incredibly simple, it makes an excellent pareve dessert, it pleases the pickiest eaters, and it is – dare I say? – pretty healthy!"

Makes 4 servings

1¾ cups dairy-free chocolate chips
5 tablespoons nondairy milk
1 tablespoon vanilla (you can also use peppermint, orange, hazelnut, etc.)
16 ounces silken tofu

Melt the chocolate chips with the nondairy milk and vanilla in a double boiler.

Process the tofu in a food processor until smooth. Add the chocolate mixture to the tofu and blend until fully combined. Refrigerate until ready to serve.

TIPS & TRICKS:

- I like to serve this dessert in crystal goblets.
- Try it topped with chopped nuts, candy canes, a cookie, or enjoy it plain.
- My credit goes to Elisa Giommi of Groton, Connecticut, and the Puritan and Genesta natural foods market of Mystic, Connecticut.

SUTLACH (SEPHARDIC RICE PUDDING)

Leatrice Gutmann

"This is my Aunt Mary Capeloto's recipe. She was a fabulous Sephardic cook. Everything she made was delicious and picture perfect. She put on a series of Sephardic cooking classes at the request of the Seattle Repertory Organization. I was her assistant – my job was to hand her whatever she needed! She taught my cousins and me how to make traditional dishes, and we continue to keep her recipes alive."

Makes 4 servings

¼ cup rice flour
¼ cup sugar
2 cups whole milk
1 teaspoon vanilla
Cinnamon, as a garnish

In a saucepan, combine the rice flour, sugar, and milk. Cook over medium-high heat, stirring constantly, until the mixture thickens. Stir in the vanilla and pour the pudding into custard cups. Sprinkle with cinnamon and refrigerate the pudding. Serve cold.

MY MOTHER'S RICE PUDDING

Daisy Israel

"My mother, Gentil Levy Israel, always said, 'My life began when I married and moved into the home of the Israel family.' Her mother died when she was an infant, and she also lost a sister and her father at an early age. Marriage brought her the large extended family she had always yearned for. Along with that, she learned how to be a wonderful homemaker and cook. This particular recipe was her own invention; besides being delicious, it fills the kitchen with a sweet aroma. We loved eating it warm from the baking dish."

Makes 6 to 8 servings

1 cup uncooked rice
6 cups warm water
4 cups milk, divided
2 eggs, beaten
1 cup sugar
Handful of raisins or dried cranberries (optional)
Cinnamon, as a garnish

Preheat the oven to 350°.

Mix the rice and warm water in a 9x13-inch glass baking dish or 3½ to 4 quart casserole dish. Bake until all the water is absorbed.

Add 2 cups of the milk to the rice. In a mixing bowl, combine the remaining 2 cups of the milk, eggs, and sugar. Add the raisins or cranberries, if desired, and pour the mixture over the rice.

Sprinkle the top of the rice pudding with cinnamon. Bake for 1 hour. Serve it warm, or refrigerate for later.

BURMUELOS

Katherine Scharhon

Makes 24 to 36 donuts

2 packages active dry yeast
4 cups warm water
2 tablespoons sugar
1 teaspoon salt
2 tablespoons vegetable oil, plus more for frying
6½ cups flour
Honey, for drizzling

Combine the yeast, 1 cup of the water, and sugar in a large bowl. Let it stand for 5 to 10 minutes, until foam forms. Add the salt, oil, remaining 3 cups water, and flour. Mix well to make a smooth, sticky dough. Cover with plastic wrap or a clean tea towel and let it rise in a warm place for 1 to 2 hours. The longer it rests, the better.

In a deep saucepan, heat the oil to 375°. With moist hands, break off 2 inch balls of dough and poke a hole in the center with your thumb or finger and drop into the hot oil (4 to 6 at a time, depending on the size of the saucepan). Flip when golden brown on the bottom. Remove with a slotted spoon when golden brown on both sides and drain on paper towels. Serve with warm honey.

TIPS & TRICKS:

- In a large plastic bag with an ample amount of cinnamon-sugar or powdered sugar, add the drained donuts. Shake vigorously to cover completely. Serve warm.

FRUIT CRISP

Laura Stusser-McNeil

"I come from a long line of berry pickers. I started as a little girl in various blackberry patches known only to my grandmothers and parents around Three Tree Point and Mercer Island. My mom always made a cobbler – not a pie – out of those precious berries and we adored it. In recent years, my mom, sisters and I have all moved on to crisps. We each have our own variation of this fast, flexible, and delicious dessert. This recipe is my version with a nod to Heidi Rabel's, What to Fix For Dinner cookbook."

Serves 10 to 12

Filling:
5 to 6 cups fresh fruit (blackberries, raspberries, blueberries, strawberries, rhubarb, sliced peaches, apples, or any combination of fruits)
1 tablespoon lemon juice
1 teaspoon lemon zest
2 cups sugar (or less, some of the berries don't need that much sugar)

Grease a 9x13-inch baking dish (that you'll want to serve from later).

Put the fruit in a large bowl and sprinkle with the lemon juice. Gently toss the fruit with the lemon zest and sugar and pour into the prepared baking dish.

Topping:
½ cup brown sugar
½ cup oats
½ cup flour
3 tablespoons butter, melted
Dash of salt
Dash of cinnamon (optional)

Vanilla ice cream, for serving

Preheat the oven to 425°.

Mix the brown sugar, oats, and flour together then add the melted butter. Mix with your fingers until crumbly and sprinkle on top of the fruit, pressing down gently.

Bake for 15 minutes then reduce the heat to 350° and bake for 30 to 40 minutes, until the topping is brown and the fruit is bubbling at the edges. Serve warm or at room temperature with vanilla ice cream.

PAPU'S POACHED PEARS

Eugene Normand

"We have a large old pear tree that yields a large number of pears some years and many fewer in other years. These are winter pears with a green-gold skin and are very firm, so we had to figure out how to use them. We give quite a few away to friends, co-workers, or shelters, but I also developed a recipe for poaching them and freezing them afterwards. It is based on a recipe I found in a cookbook, but I modified it, because the original was far too sweet."

Serves 12 to 16

6 to 8 medium to large pears, peeled
1 cup red or white wine
1/3 cup sugar
1/2 teaspoon lemon juice
1 cinnamon stick

Cut the pears into quarters, removing the seeds, seed membranes, and stems.

In a large pot, bring the wine, sugar, lemon juice, and cinnamon stick to a boil. Add some of the pear pieces to the sauce (in a single layer) and keep the mixture boiling with the pot covered.

After 2 to 3 minutes, turn the pear pieces over and check the firmness of the pieces with a fork. When the pieces feel firm, yet soft to the touch of a fork, transfer to a bowl. Repeat this process until all the pear pieces are poached, keeping in mind the poaching time depends on the ripeness of the pears to start.

When all the pieces have been poached, pour any remaining sauce over the completed pears.

TIPS & TRICKS:

- After cooling the pears, they can be frozen.
- If using a plastic storage container, keep it covered while the pears cool and wipe away the condensation that accumulates on the lid before freezing.

STONE FRUIT DESSERT

Darcy Goodman

Serves 8 to 10

6 pieces stone fruit, pitted, cut into sixths, and pricked
½ lime, juiced
3 tablespoons sugar or Splenda®
2 tablespoons butter
2 sprigs fresh rosemary
Vanilla ice cream, for serving

Preheat the oven to 400°.

Put the fruit pieces into a 9x13-inch baking dish and sprinkle with the lime juice and sugar, then dot with the butter. Place the rosemary sprigs on top.

Bake for 20 minutes and serve warm with vanilla ice cream.

TIPS & TRICKS:

- Peaches, nectarines, and plums work well in this recipe. For plums, use a smaller baking dish or just add more plums.
- You can use one type of stone fruit or a combination of many.

STRAWBERRY FLUFF

Beverly Grashin

"A fabulous dessert after a heavy meal. A family favorite at Seder."

Serves 6

2 egg whites, stiffly beaten
1 cup sugar
1 tablespoon lemon juice
1½ cups fresh strawberries, mashed
4 ounces chocolate, melted (optional)

Prepare 6 individual custard cups or ramekins by lining each with plastic wrap.

Beat the egg whites until stiff, gradually adding the sugar. Add the lemon juice and continue beating. Fold in the mashed strawberries. Pour into individual custard cups or ramekins and freeze until hard. Unmold when frozen and dip into the melted and cooled chocolate. Refreeze until ready to serve.

TIPS & TRICKS:

- To melt the chocolate, microwave it with just a touch of canola oil in 30-second increments, stirring after each interval, until the chocolate is melted and smooth. Cool.

Old Cakes, New Cakes, Plum Cakes, Cheesecakes

Not only are our cake recipes rich with butter, oil, eggs, and sugar; they are likewise laden with emotions and memories, nearly every one metaphorically rich, light, and sweet all at once.

More explicitly than any other chapter, these recipes span generations and continents. Amanda Azous recounts her mother's survival through the Holocaust and resettlement in Seattle, and Susie Sherman describes the cake that originated in 1914 and became the ubiquitous "holiday cake" among her surviving family from former Czechoslovakia.

Jane Preuss' and Doris Stiefel's plum cake recipes both convey the sweetness of confections as they were prepared on the cusp of tragic change for European Jewry. In a letter from July 5, 1939, Jane Preuss' grandmother, Mitzi, in Austria, wrote to her daughter in America about impending changes and her fears of having to leave her home and her friends. Alas, she must close, she says, as she has to tend to a cherry strudel. Then she will go for into town for some fresh air. Imagining the dough on the counter as Mitzi strolled into a warm sunny Austrian afternoon in 1939 makes the reader ache to be able to reach through the letter and pull her and her strudel to safety.

But not all stories are so weighty. Joan Lerner recalls not being allowed to touch the banana nut cake until all her mother's Canasta friends had taken their shares, and Joan Alhadeff meditates on her boys becoming men, but always coming back to her applesauce cake. Diane Douglas wistfully writes about making her grandmother's Depression-era Poor Man's Cake when she misses home and her parents. Marilyn Sidel recalls the annual ritual of the Olympia Jewish community calling her mother the week before Passover to get her "never fail" Passover cake, which from year to year they never failed to forget. Julia Niebuhr Eulenberg humorously reflects on the riddle that emerged from her grandmother's Romanian accent: "When is a cake not a cake?" See her recipe for the answer (page 272)!

Given the powerful memories associated with cake, it comes as no surprise that the vast majority of recipes we received were for desserts. The apparent theme is the lasting emotional and familial attachment to a good dessert. Doris Stiefel ponders the lineage of her plum cake and meditates on its continuation through her own grandchildren, who love picking plums from the tree she and her husband planted when they built their home together many years ago.

TIDBIT:
The history of cheesecake goes beyond New York's famous. In fact, cheesecake was known to the ancient Greeks and Romans, who concocted a dish out of cheese, flour, and honey and offered it to the gods. A recipe for a sweet "tarte of chese" also appears in the 16th-century cookbook, *A Proper newe Booke of Cokerye.*

OLD CAKES, NEW CAKES, PLUM CAKES, CHEESECAKES

GRANDMA MARY'S HONEY CAKE

Lucy Friedman

"I received this recipe from my mother-in-law, Mary Friedman."

Serves 12 to 16

4 eggs
1½ cups sugar
1 cup honey
1 cup oil
1 cup warm brewed strong coffee
3½ cups flour, sifted
2 teaspoons baking soda
1 teaspoon ginger
1 teaspoon ground cloves
1 whole lemon, ground in food processor

Preheat the oven to 350°. Grease and flour a 10x15-inch pan.

Cream together the eggs and sugar in a large bowl. Add the honey, oil, and coffee. In a separate bowl, sift the flour with the baking soda, ginger, and cloves, and add to the wet ingredients. Add the ground lemon. Pour the mixture into the pan and bake for 65 minutes.

TIPS & TRICKS:

- ½ cup dark raisins, walnuts, or both can be added to the batter before pouring it into the pan.

"Our honey cake recipe came from our Aunt Anna who served it on Rosh Hashanah and Yom Kippur. Aunt Anna was a wonderful cook. She and Uncle Dave lived in a small apartment with a tiny kitchen and a huge dining room. No one could fit in the kitchen to help Aunt Anna with her scrumptious holiday meals, so she cooked and served and cooked and served some more. Everyone enjoyed the heavenly food she prepared and would plead with her to come to the table to sit and eat. Still she cooked and served. When finally the last of the food was on the table she would sit down to eat. Everyone around her was completely satiated from the delicious feast they had enjoyed. Aunt Anna would look around and ask 'So, how come no one's eating?'"

~ Nancy Corning and Karen Israel

RACHEL'S HONEY CAKE

Katherine Zinger Miller

"Memories of eating my grandmother's honey cake are sweet, just like this cake, because my grandmother was like a second mother to me. I remember watching her make this in her kitchen every Rosh Hashanah. She was from St. Petersburg, Russia, and immigrated to Montreal, Quebec, in 1978."

Serves 12 to 16

3½ cups all-purpose flour
2 teaspoons baking powder
1 teaspoon baking soda
4 teaspoons ground cinnamon
1 cup vegetable oil
1 cup honey
1 cup sugar
1 cup brown sugar
3 large eggs, room temperature
1 teaspoon vanilla
1 cup Coca-Cola® (diet or regular)
½ cup orange juice, freshly squeezed
¼ cup whiskey

Preheat the oven to 350°. Generously grease a 9x13-inch pan or a 10-inch tube pan. For the tube pan, line the bottom with lightly greased parchment paper, cut to fit.

In a large bowl, whisk together the flour, baking powder, baking soda, and cinnamon. Add the oil, honey, sugar, brown sugar, eggs, vanilla, cola, orange juice, and whiskey.

Using a strong wire whisk or in an electric mixer on a slow speed, stir together the ingredients to form a thick, well-blended batter, making sure that no ingredients are stuck to the bottom.

Spoon the batter into the prepared pan. Bake until the cake springs back when you gently touch the cake center, about 40 to 45 minutes for the 9x13-inch pan or 1 hour to 1¼ hours for the tube pan.

POOR MAN'S CAKE

Diane Douglas

"This recipe comes from my grandmother, Anna, and I understand she enjoyed making it for her son-in-law, my dad. Although my grandmother died when I was very young, this cake became a mainstay in my parents' house. There was always an extra one kept in the freezer in the cellar in case guests showed up unexpectedly and needed to be fed. Frequently, it was our breakfast on Shabbat morning. After I left home, I started making the cake and sweetly, it became a favorite of my father-in-law. My mother and I enjoyed making it for him just as my grandmother had shown her affection for my dad by making it for him. I make this cake when I miss home and when I think of my parents. I copied the recipe and gave it to all my friends who came to visit during my mother's shiva. I am told it is called a Poor Man's Cake because it contains no eggs –an expensive luxury during the Depression."

Serves 12 to 16

2 cups raisins
2 cups sugar
2 cups water
¾ cup canola oil
2 teaspoons cinnamon
1 teaspoon ground cloves
1 teaspoon salt
2 teaspoons baking soda
3½ cups flour

Preheat the oven to 350°. Lightly grease and flour a 9x13-inch pan.

In a large saucepan, combine the raisins, sugar, water, oil, cinnamon, cloves, and salt. Bring to a boil and cook for 3 minutes. When slightly cooled, dissolve the baking soda with just a bit of water to make a paste, and add to the batter. Gradually add the flour and mix well.

Pour into the pan and bake for 35 minutes, until the top springs back when lightly touched.

HOLIDAY CAKE

Susie Sherman

"My immediate family of four, my mother Emmy, my father Rudi, my sister Eva, and I, came to America in October of 1943. My family was from Czechoslovakia. I use the term 'my family of four' because the rest of this large, dear, extended family who stayed in Czechoslovakia did not survive. After several stops, the four of us luckily made our way to England, and from there, America. My mother was an excellent baker and enjoyed making wonderful sweet treats for us. Her family made this cake in Europe, but it was made for special occasions growing up. It was a given that the Holiday Cake was served for special occasions such as birthdays and other holidays. The cake is flourless and can also be used for Passover. A cake was considered fancy and special if it was made without flour. This recipe was originated in 1914 by a chef to commemorate the opening of the Panama Canal and was called the Panamatorte. My mother, Emmy Rindler, changed it and treated our family to it on special occasions. Our family called it Holiday Cake. I changed her recipe for my taste, and this is the version that I make."

Makes one 2-layer cake

11 eggs, separated
1 cup sugar
1 cup semisweet chocolate chips
2 cups walnuts, ground

Preheat the oven to 325°. Line two 9-inch springform pans with parchment paper and lightly grease the pans.

Beat the egg whites until very stiff, then refrigerate. In a separate bowl, beat the egg yolks and sugar well. Melt the chocolate chips, cool, and blend them into the beaten egg yolks. Stir in the ground walnuts.

Gently fold the chocolate mixture into the egg whites. Pour half of the batter into each of the springform pans. Bake for 25 minutes. The cake is done when an inserted toothpick comes out fairly clean. Let the layers cool completely.

Filling and Icing:
1 cup unsalted butter, softened
1¼ cups powdered sugar, or to taste
1 teaspoon vanilla
Dash of rum
1½ cups semisweet chocolate chips, or to taste, melted

Cream the butter. Add the powdered sugar, vanilla, and rum and beat until well blended. Mix in the chocolate chips. Use the frosting as a filling between the layers, and icing on the sides and the top. Keep the cake in the refrigerator, or freeze for later.

> *"My honey cake recipe was given to me by Pearl Singer who was born and raised in the Spokane Jewish community. Pearl used to bring her honey cake to the weekly Kiddush lunch that we have after Shabbat morning services at Temple Beth Shalom. My mom usually made this cake in a Bundt pan, but sometimes in loaves. It was always moist and yummy."*
>
> ~ Mary Noble

MARGE'S NEVER FAIL PASSOVER CAKE

Marilyn Sidel

"This was my mother's recipe. I don't know where she got it, but it was renamed 'Marge's Never Fail Passover Cake.' I have fond memories of the phone ringing the week before Passover, when the women of our small congregation in Olympia called to ask for the recipe – every year! No one ever saved it from year to year. It turned into our private joke and always gave us a big laugh."

Serves 12 to 14

12 eggs, separated
⅓ cup Passover cake meal
½ cup potato starch
2 cups sugar
1 lemon, rind grated (optional)
2 tablespoons lemon juice (optional)

Preheat the oven to 350°.

In an electric mixer, beat the egg whites until stiff and dry. Gradually add the sugar, one tablespoon at a time, beating constantly.

In a small bowl, mix the cake meal and the potato starch together. Fold them into the egg whites on low speed.

TIPS & TRICKS:

- If your eggs are especially large, the cake often rises way above the top of the tube pan during baking. I put the upside-down tube pan on a 1-quart pop bottle while the cake is cooling.

In another small bowl, beat the egg yolks until they are lemon colored. Add the lemon rind and lemon juice, if desired. Fold the yolks into the egg white mixture.

Pour the batter into an ungreased 12-inch tube pan. Bake for 1 hour and 10 minutes.

Cool the cake upside down before removing it from the pan.

PASSOVER NUT CAKE

Julia Niebuhr Eulenberg

"This recipe has been handed down from Sarah Rosenthal Esac, grandmother of Michael Eulenberg, and great-grandmother of Rabbi Sarah Rubin and Eric Eulenberg. Grandma Esac's Romanian accent paved the way for a family riddle invented by her son-in-law. When the grandchildren asked what was she baking, Grandma Esac replied, 'a not cake.' Ed Eulenberg's riddle? 'When is a cake not a cake?' The answer, of course, is when it is a 'not cake' – or this very fine and moist Passover Nut Cake."

Serves 12

10 large eggs, separated and room temperature
1½ cups sugar
1 medium orange, juiced and finely zested
½ lemon, finely zested
1 medium apple, grated
¾ cup Passover cake meal, sifted
¼ cup potato starch, sifted
1 cup walnuts or pecans, finely chopped

Preheat the oven to 325°.

Beat the egg whites until stiff and foamy. In a separate bowl, beat the egg yolks until thick and lemony in color. Slowly add the sugar to the egg yolks. Add the orange juice, orange rind, lemon rind, and the grated apple. Then add the cake meal and the potato starch. Fold in the nuts, and then fold in the stiff egg whites.

Bake for 60 minutes in an ungreased 10-inch tube sponge cake pan. When baked, turn the cake pan upside down over the neck of a wine bottle to cool completely. Don't worry, the cake will not fall out of the pan.

APPLE CAKE FOR THE NEW YEAR

Cynthia Flash Hemphill

"This apple cake is a Rosh Hashanah favorite, but you can make it any time of the year. Be sure to hand mix the batter in a large bowl because it is very thick and bulky and takes a lot of muscle to mix. It bakes up very moist, with a hard meringue-like crust on top and will store for at least a week in the refrigerator."

Serves 12 to 15

3 cups sugar
1 tablespoon baking soda
1½ teaspoons cinnamon
1¼ teaspoons salt
¾ cup vegetable oil
3 eggs
1½ teaspoons vanilla
6 cups tart apples, peeled, cored, and sliced (or chunked)
1½ cups walnuts, coarsely chopped
3 cups flour

Preheat the oven to 325°. Grease a 9x13-inch metal pan or if you prefer to use a glass dish, reduce the oven temperature to 300°.

In a large bowl, combine the sugar, baking soda, cinnamon, salt, oil, eggs, and vanilla. Add the apples and walnuts and stir until just covered with the batter. Stir in the flour.

Pour the batter into the pan. Bake the cake for 1 hour and 20 minutes. The cake will be cooked when a toothpick comes out clean. You may have to bake the cake up to 15 to 20 minutes longer, so check every 5 minutes. When done, remove the cake from the oven and cool in the pan on a wire rack. When cooled, cut into desired size squares.

TIPS & TRICKS:

- This apple cake is delicious when served just plain, but if you prefer, serve it with caramel sauce drizzled on the plate with a dollop of whipped cream.

ALMOND POPPY SEED CAKE WITH ORANGE GLAZE

Robyn Anderson

"My mom and I are always baking in the kitchen! She is a fabulous baker, and I have learned everything I know from experimenting in the kitchen with her over the years. To keep things interesting, we are always trying new recipes. Of course we have our favorites, and growing up I can remember making the classics from apple pie, to decorative cookies, to delicious brownies. This cake was always one of my favorites, as I loved the almond flavor and the sweetness from the orange glaze. Every year I would request this cake for my birthday."

Serves 8

2¾ cups sugar
1 cup oil
3 large eggs
1½ teaspoons vanilla
1 teaspoon almond extract
3 cups all-purpose flour
2 tablespoons poppy seeds
1½ teaspoons baking powder
½ teaspoon salt
1½ cups milk

Preheat the oven to 350°. Grease and flour a 12-cup Bundt pan.

Using an electric mixer, mix the sugar, oil, eggs, vanilla, and almond extract until well combined. In a medium bowl, mix together the flour, poppy seeds, baking powder, and salt. Stir the dry ingredients into the sugar mixture, alternating with the milk, beginning and ending with the dry ingredients.

Pour the batter into the prepared pan. Bake for 50 to 55 minutes, until a tester inserted near the center of the cake comes out clean. Cool the cake in the pan for 10 minutes.

Glaze:
1 cup powdered sugar
¼ cup orange juice
¼ teaspoon almond extract

To make the glaze, whisk the powdered sugar, orange juice, and almond extract in a small bowl until blended.

Turn the cake out onto a cooling rack on top of a baking sheet. Poke small holes on top of the cake and spoon the glaze over the warm cake, allowing the glaze to run down the sides of the cake. Continue to scoop up the extra glaze on the baking sheet and pour it over the cake.

Cool the cake completely and serve.

SUNNY 7-UP® CAKE

Cindy Masin

"A friend from North Carolina gave me this recipe long ago. Her son was living in Seattle at the time and was celebrating his birthday. Since she could not be here, she asked me to make the cake and take it to her son. I had never made it before, but I haven't stopped making it since. It's simple to make; it's rich, buttery, and perfect all on its own, but with fresh berries of any kind, it is truly scrumptious."

Serves 12 to16

1½ cups butter, softened
3 cups sugar
5 eggs
3 cups flour
2 tablespoons lemon extract
¾ cup 7-UP®

Preheat the oven to 325°. Grease and flour a Bundt pan.

In a large bowl, cream the butter and sugar together. Add the eggs and beat until fluffy. Add the flour, lemon extract, and 7-UP®.

Pour the mixture into the prepared pan. Bake for 1 hour to 1 hour and 10 minutes, until the top springs back when touched. Cool the cake in the pan for 20 minutes before removing to a wire rack.

Glaze:
½ cup powdered sugar
Lemon juice

While the cake is cooking, mix the powdered sugar and lemon juice to make the glaze. Once the cake is moved to the wire rack, immediately drizzle the glaze over the cake.

TIPS & TRICKS:

- This cake can be frozen and enjoyed later.

APPLESAUCE CAKE WITH MAPLE BUTTERCREAM FROSTING

Joan Alhadeff

"The aroma of apples, spices, and maple bring warmth and a sense that 'all is well' as each of my three guys came through the door. My silent way of saying, 'I love you.' Just as an empty cake pan with a few crumbs, smashed raisins, and icing smears was a silent confirmation stating, 'Love you too.'

"I found it hard to transition from 'mommy' to 'mom' as my adolescent sons seemed to be coming and going and not needing me so much. Baking was something I loved to do, and they seemed to appreciate so much. This cake is the one they still remember."

Serves 12 to 15

2½ cups flour
1½ teaspoons baking soda
¾ teaspoon baking powder
1½ teaspoons ginger
1½ teaspoons cinnamon
1½ teaspoons nutmeg
½ teaspoon salt
½ cup butter, softened
1¼ cups sugar
1½ cups unsweetened applesauce
2 large eggs
½ cup raisins
⅔ cup walnuts, chopped

Preheat the oven to 350°. Grease a 9x13-inch pan.

Sift together the flour, baking soda, baking powder, ginger, cinnamon, nutmeg, and salt. Set aside.

In a mixer, cream the butter and the sugar. Add the applesauce and then the eggs. Mix in the dry ingredients until just incorporated. Fold in the raisins and the nuts.

Pour the mixture into the prepared pan. Bake for 30 to 35 minutes, until a toothpick inserted into the center comes out clean. Cool completely before frosting.

Frosting:
3 cups powdered sugar
⅓ cup butter
½ cup maple syrup

Mix the powdered sugar, butter, and maple syrup together and beat until smooth.

WESTHAVEN CAKE

Cindy Stratiner

"We used to go to visit Grandma Rosie often and she almost always had this cake around for us. It was a favorite treat for us (and for her card and Mahjongg ladies). We would joke with her about how much we loved her 'crummy' cake, as when we were finished there were always chocolate crumbs all over the table and the floor. Grandma was maybe 4'11" and so much fun to be around. She loved to see us smile and laugh, and she always had tissues up her sleeve in case we had the sniffles. Besides feeding us cake, she loved to play with us; hide and seek when we were young, and then it was on to all the card games that she could teach us. Grandpa would read to us or take us to the park when Grandma needed a rest. We always had a wonderful time at our Grandma Rose and Grandpa Sid's home."

Serves 8 to 10

½ cup dates, pitted and chopped
1 teaspoon baking soda
1 cup boiling water
1 cup shortening
2 eggs
1 cup sugar
1¾ cups flour
3 heaping tablespoons cocoa powder
½ teaspoon vanilla
½ teaspoon peppermint extract
½ cup chocolate chips

Preheat the oven to 350°. Grease a 9x13-inch baking dish.

Mix dates, baking soda, and water in a small bowl and let cool.

In a large bowl, mix the shortening, eggs, sugar, flour, cocoa powder, vanilla, peppermint extract, and chocolate chips, and fold in the date mixture.

Topping:
½ cup chocolate chips
½ cup almonds, chopped
¼ cup mint chips

In a small bowl, mix the chocolate chips, almonds, and mint chips.

Pour the batter into the baking dish. Sprinkle the topping mixture over the batter.

Bake for 35 to 45 minutes. Cool on a rack.

BLIND DATE CAKE

Michele Keller

"This recipe was handed down from my mother, Jeanette Galanti. We ate it before the meal to break the fast after Yom Kippur."

Serves 12 to 18

1 cup dates, chopped
1 teaspoon baking soda
1½ cups boiling water
½ cup shortening
1 cup sugar
2 eggs
1 teaspoon vanilla
1½ cups flour
½ teaspoon salt
¾ teaspoon baking soda

Preheat the oven to 350°. Grease a 9x13-inch pan.

Combine the dates and baking soda in a medium bowl. Pour the boiling water over the date mixture and let it stand for 5 minutes.

In an electric mixer, cream the shortening and 1 cup of the sugar. Add the eggs and vanilla.

In a separate bowl, combine the flour, salt, and baking soda. Alternately, add the flour mixture and the date mixture to the shortening mixture. Beat for 3 minutes. Pour the cake batter into the prepared pan.

Topping:
½ cup sugar
½ cup walnuts, chopped
1 cup semisweet or bittersweet chocolate chips

In a small mixing bowl, combine the sugar, walnuts, and chocolate chips. Sprinkle the topping over the cake and bake for 35 to 40 minutes.

PUMPKIN CHOCOLATE CHIP SPICE CAKE

Gloria Bensussen and Shelley Bensussen

Serves 8

½ cup butter
1¼ cups sugar
2 eggs
2¼ cups self-rising flour
¼ teaspoon salt
1 teaspoon ground ginger
1 teaspoon ground nutmeg
¾ cup milk
1 cup pumpkin purée
¼ teaspoon baking soda
1 12-ounce bag semisweet chocolate chips

Preheat the oven to 350°. Grease 9-inch square cake pan.

Cream the butter and sugar until light and fluffy, adding the eggs, one at a time. In a separate bowl sift together the flour, salt, ginger, and nutmeg. In a third bowl, combine the milk, pumpkin, and baking soda. Add the flour and pumpkin mixture alternately to the creamed mixture, making sure each is well blended before adding the next. Stir in the chocolate chips.

Pour the batter into the prepared pan and bake for 50 to 55 minutes, until a toothpick inserted in center comes out clean.

CAKE FOR THE BOYS' BIRTHDAY

Debra Schwartz

Serves 8 to 12

7 eggs, separated
½ cup hot water
1 teaspoon vanilla
2 cups sugar
2 cups flour
½ teaspoon salt
1 teaspoon cream of tartar
Whipped cream, for serving

Preheat the oven to 250°. Grease a tube pan.

Beat the egg yolks until thick. Add the hot water and vanilla and beat for an additional 5 minutes.

Sift the flour and sugar 6 times. When completed, fold the flour mixture into the yolk mixture.

Beat the egg whites and salt until foamy, then add the cream of tartar and beat until stiff. Fold into the egg yolk-flour mixture and pour into the prepared pan.

Bake for 35 minutes, then increase the oven temperature to 300° and bake for 15 minutes, then increase the oven temperature to 325° and bake for a final 30 minutes. Cool and serve with whipped cream.

CLASSIC BANANA CAKE

Cindy Masin

"We went to a wedding many years ago in San Francisco. The banana wedding cake that was served was very moist, dense, full of flavor, yet still old-fashioned...the best I had ever tasted. After many tries, I finally found a banana cake recipe that fits that bill perfectly. It's a classic."

Serves 12 to 16

3 cups all-purpose flour
2 teaspoons baking soda
½ teaspoon salt
1 cup unsalted butter
2 cups sugar
2 teaspoons vanilla
2 large eggs, room temperature
1½ to 1¾ cups bananas, very ripe (about 4 bananas)
1 cup sour cream

Preheat the oven to 350°. Generously butter three 9-inch layer pans and line the pans with parchment rounds.

In a bowl, whisk the flour, baking soda, and salt together and set aside.

Using an electric mixer, cream the butter and sugar. Beat in the vanilla, then add the eggs, one at a time, beating for about 1 minute after each egg has been added. Reduce the mixer speed to low and mix in the bananas. Finally, mix in half of the flour mixture (don't be disturbed if the batter curdles), sour cream, and then the rest of the flour mixture. Distribute the batter evenly into the pans, tap the pans on the counter to release any bubbles, and smooth the top.

Bake for approximately 25 minutes, until a thin knife inserted deep into the center of the cake comes out clean and the cake bounces back when touched in the middle. Cool completely on racks then remove from pans.

Buttercream Frosting:
6 cups powdered sugar
2 teaspoons vanilla
¾ cup butter, softened
5 to 6 tablespoons milk

Beat the sugar, vanilla, and butter with an electric mixer. Slowly add the milk until the desired consistency then beat for two minutes, scraping the bowl often. Use the frosting as a filling between the layers, and icing on the sides and the top.

MOTHER'S BANANA NUT CAKE

Joan Lerner

"Della Tall loved her friends and the Canasta game. Mother would always have bananas ripening to 'perfection' in the kitchen for her cake. My brother, Leonard, and I were forbidden to eat the special bananas as they were for 'the cake.' We were not allowed any until after the ladies had their share and took pieces home to their husbands."

Serves 10 to 14

1½ cups sugar
½ cup butter
2 eggs, beaten
1¾ cups flour
1½ teaspoons baking powder
1 teaspoon baking soda
Pinch of salt
5 tablespoons buttermilk (or sour milk)
2 large, well-ripened bananas, mashed
1 teaspoon vanilla
1 cup nuts, chopped

Preheat the oven to 350°. Grease and flour two 9-inch baking pans.

Cream the butter and sugar in a large bowl. Add the eggs.

Sift the flour, baking powder, baking soda, and salt together. Add the flour mixture alternately with the buttermilk to the creamed butter. Add the bananas, vanilla, and nuts.

Pour the batter into the baking pans. Bake for 35 to 40 minutes. Cool completely before frosting with your favorite icing.

CARROT CAKE

Andrea Lott

Serves 16

3 cups unbleached all-purpose flour
2¼ cups sugar
1 teaspoon salt
1 tablespoon baking soda
1 tablespoon ground cinnamon
1 cup vegetable oil
½ cup unsweetened applesauce
4 large eggs, lightly beaten
1 tablespoon vanilla
1½ cups walnuts, chopped
1½ cups shredded sweetened coconut
5 cups carrots, grated (about 6 to 8 carrots)
¾ cups crushed pineapple, drained
¾ to 1 cup raisins

Preheat the oven to 350°. Grease two 9-inch cake pans.

Sift the flour, sugar, salt, baking soda, and cinnamon into a large bowl. Add the oil, applesauce, eggs, and vanilla. Beat well. Fold in the walnuts, coconut, carrots, pineapple, and raisins.

Divide the batter between the prepared pans and smooth the tops with a rubber spatula. Set on the middle rack of the oven and bake for about 50 minutes, until the edges have pulled away from the sides and a cake tester inserted in the center comes out clean.

Cool the cakes for 15 minutes, and then remove them from the cake pans and cool completely on a wire rack, at least 3 hours. Frost with cream cheese frosting.

Frosting:
1 8-ounce package cream cheese, softened
4 tablespoons unsalted butter, room temperature
3 cups powdered sugar, sifted
1 teaspoon vanilla
½ lemon, juiced (optional)

Cream the cream cheese and butter in the bowl of an electric mixture. Add the powdered sugar and continue beating until fully incorporated; the mixture should be free of lumps. Stir in the vanilla and lemon juice, if desired.

MY NEW FAVORITE COCONUT CAKE

Diane Cheifetz

"My favorite cake for years and years has been a coconut cake from the Jewish Day School cookbook. It was made with a packaged yellow cake mix. But, for my last birthday, my sister made this delicious coconut cake from scratch, so from now on, I'll be requesting that one instead. It is best with cream cheese frosting then covered with coconut or even toasted coconut. Either way, you can't go wrong."

Serves 12 to 15

1½ cups unsalted butter, room temperature, plus extra for greasing the pans
2 cups sugar
5 extra-large eggs, room temperature
2 teaspoons vanilla
1 teaspoon almond extract
3 cups all-purpose flour, plus extra for dusting pans
1 teaspoon baking powder
½ teaspoon baking soda
½ teaspoon kosher salt
1 cup buttermilk
6 ounces sweetened shredded coconut

Preheat the oven to 350°. Grease two 9-inch round cake pans, then line them with parchment rounds. Grease the parchment paper, and then dust lightly with flour.

In the bowl of an electric mixer, cream the butter and sugar on medium-high speed until light yellow and fluffy, about 5 minutes.

Crack the eggs into a small bowl. Turn the mixer to medium and add the eggs, one at a time, scraping down the bowl only once during mixing. Add the vanilla and almond extracts and mix well. Don't be concerned if the mixture curdles.

In a separate bowl, sift together the flour, baking powder, baking soda, and salt. With the mixer on low, alternatively add the flour mixture and buttermilk in three parts, beginning and ending with the flour mixture. Mix until just combined. Fold in the coconut with a rubber spatula.

Pour the batter evenly into the 2 pans and smooth the top. Bake in the center of the oven for 45 to 55 minutes, until the tops are brown and a cake tester comes out clean. Cool on a wire rack for 30 minutes, and then remove the cakes to the rack until completely cool. Frost with the cream cheese frosting and decorate with the coconut.

Cream Cheese Frosting:
2 8-ounce packages cream cheese, softened
1 cup unsalted butter, room temperature
¾ teaspoon vanilla
¼ teaspoon almond extract
1 pound powdered sugar

6 ounces sweetened shredded coconut, for decorating

In the bowl of an electric mixer, combine the cream cheese, butter, vanilla, and almond extract on low speed. Add the powdered sugar and mix until smooth.

To assemble the cake, place one layer on a cake plate, rounded-side down, and spread with frosting. Place the second layer on top, rounded-side up, and frost the top and sides. Sprinkle with coconut on the top and press more coconut onto the sides.

TIPS & TRICKS:

❖ To toast the coconut, place it on parchment paper-lined baking sheet and put in a 350° oven for 7 to 10 minutes, until golden brown, stirring occasionally. Watch carefully as the coconut can go from golden to burnt in a very short period of time. Pat the coconut onto the cake.

MOM'S MARBLE CAKE

Amanda Azous

"Paula Azous was born Peenya Priseler in Felshiu Visou, Romania, on April 25, 1928, to Bella and Hannan Priseler. She survived the Nazi concentration camps and afterward met Mordahi Azous, a Greek Jew from Solonika, in a Liberation Camp. Like many young people who suffered from the Nazis and survived, they quickly found each other, got married, and tried to make a normal life for themselves back in Salonika. As a result, Paula became an expert cook in both Ashkenazic and Sephardic cooking. Her legacy of culinary delights has left children and grandchildren hungering for her scrumptious dinners and unique desserts since she passed away in 2007.

"Paula always kept her recipes secret, and they were not written down. Once a friend of hers, Vefa Alexiadou, a famous cook and cookbook writer from Salonika, came to visit Paula in Seattle, where she lived the latter half of her life. Vefa documented as many recipes as she could. This recipe of mom's that we are happy to share is called Mom's Marble Cake, and there is really none that compares. It is a dry cake with a moist chocolate center and not too sweet. It can even be made with matzo meal (sans flour and baking powder) for a perfect Pesach dessert. It is our pleasure to share this old family recipe with you."

Serves 10 to 12

½ cup butter
1¼ cups sugar
3 teaspoons vanilla
8 eggs
2 cups flour
2 teaspoons baking powder
1½ cups walnuts, finely chopped
2 tablespoons cocoa powder
Powdered sugar, for dusting

Preheat the oven to 350°. Grease and flour a Bundt pan.

Cream the butter and 1 cup of the sugar together in a large bowl. Add the vanilla and eggs. Gradually add the flour and baking powder, and then fold in the walnuts.

Remove half of the batter and add the cocoa powder and remaining ¼ cup of the sugar to the remaining batter.

Pour the reserved batter into the prepared pan. Carefully spoon the chocolate batter into the center of the white batter.

Bake for 1 hour. Dust with powdered sugar when slightly cooled.

SOLSTICE CAKE (SOUR CREAM FUDGE CAKE)

Beth Cordova

"My mother, Rose Bender, was the daughter of Russian and Romanian immigrants. She, like many of her peers, was interested in assimilating into the American melting pot – cultural hopes of education, opportunity, and promoting social justice for all. This emphasis led her away from Ashkenazic roots and rituals and drew her into many worlds – juggling work and home life, political activism, and becoming a highly regarded maker of special-occasion cakes and confections. Rose's sour cream fudge cake was always in demand among family and her many circles of friends. Delicious, durable, and a crowd pleaser, this cake became our favorite birthday and special-occasion cake.

"Our oldest son developed a passion for astronomy at about two. The first appearance of the 'Solstice Cake,' sour cream fudge cake, followed shortly. The cake was doubled in quantity, baked in a sheet pan, and all the constellations of the summer sky were added on top of the icing for decoration. Until Alan graduated from high school, the Solstice Cake would faithfully appear at large gatherings on June 21 or in the classroom close to December 21.

"It is easy to make this cake to feed 60 people! The Solstice Cake has also appeared as the high school cross-country team home running course, a giant soccer ball, a basketball court, and even as a marching band hat. Delicious! Durable! Memorable!

"My mother passed away August 23, 2010. May this recipe be accepted in her memory."

Serves 12 to 16

½ cup Dutch process cocoa powder, plus extra for dusting pan
¾ cup boiling water
½ cup butter, plus extra for greasing the pan
2 cups sugar
2 teaspoons vanilla
½ cup sour cream
½ teaspoon baking soda
2 cups cake flour, sifted
½ teaspoon salt
3 egg whites

Preheat the oven to 350°. Grease and dust two 9-inch cake pans with cocoa powder.

Add the boiling water to the cocoa powder and stir until smooth. Cool.

In a large bowl, cream the butter and sugar until well blended. Add the cooled cocoa mixture and vanilla and beat well.

In another bowl, mix the sour cream and baking soda and stir until bubbles form. Add to the cake batter and beat well.

In a small bowl, sift the flour and the salt together. Add to the cake batter and beat until smooth.

In a separate bowl, beat the egg whites until firm, but not dry. Gently fold the egg whites into the cake batter with a spoon. Pour the cake batter into the prepared pans and bake for 30 minutes.

Mocha Whipped Cream:
1 quart whipping cream
¼ cup Dutch process cocoa powder
2 teaspoons instant espresso powder
½ cup sugar
4 teaspoons vanilla
Pinch of salt

Beat the whipping cream, cocoa powder, espresso powder, sugar, vanilla, and salt. Cover and chill for 1 hour, until the whipped cream is firm.

Chocolate Frosting:
5 ounces unsweetened chocolate
5 tablespoons butter
4 cups powdered sugar
⅛ teaspoon salt
1 teaspoon instant espresso powder, dissolved in 1 teaspoon water
⅔ cup whole or 2% milk
2 teaspoons vanilla

In the top of a double boiler, melt the chocolate and butter until smooth.

With an electric mixer, beat the powdered sugar, salt, espresso, milk, and vanilla. Add the melted chocolate to the sugar mixture and blend completely. The mixture may need a bit more milk to achieve a spreading consistency.

Once the cake has cooled, split the layers, and fill with the whipped cream. Top the cake with the chocolate frosting.

TIPS & TRICKS:

- The cake may be assembled a day ahead of serving so the flavors can meld together.

> *"My mother, Shirley Teitelbaum, was noted for her outstanding cooking and baking. She was especially known for her famous chocolate cake. She so enjoyed making her cake for all generations, from her contemporaries to newlyweds. Shirley's cake was always requested for important family occasions."*
>
> ~ Frances Rogers

INCREDIBLE CHOCOLATE CAKE

Leslie Rosen

"I started making this cake for special occasions almost four decades ago. It remains a favorite of family and friends to this day."

Makes one 2-layer cake

4 squares unsweetened chocolate
2 cups flour
2 cups sugar
Pinch of salt
½ cup butter, softened
1 cup hot water
½ cup buttermilk
1½ teaspoons baking soda
2 teaspoons vanilla
2 eggs, beaten

Preheat the oven to 350°. Butter and lightly flour two 9-inch round cake pans or use parchment rounds to line the bottom of the two pans.

Melt and slightly cool the chocolate.

In the bowl of an electric mixer, blend the flour, sugar, and salt. Add the chocolate, butter, and hot water. Mix the buttermilk with the baking soda and add to the mixture. Next, add the vanilla and eggs. Beat at medium speed for 2 minutes.

Divide the mixture evenly between the two prepared pans and bake for about 30 minutes, until the cake springs back when touched in the middle.

TIPS & TRICKS:

- You can add 6 ounces of mini chocolate chips to the batter before baking, if desired.

Cool the cakes on a wire rack for 15 minutes and then remove the cakes from the pans to cool completely before frosting.

Chocolate Frosting:
½ cup butter, melted
⅔ cup unsweetened cocoa powder
3 cups powdered sugar
⅓ cup milk
1 teaspoon vanilla

Combine the butter and cocoa powder in a mixing bowl. Alternately, add the powdered sugar and milk, beating on medium speed to a spreadable consistency. Add the vanilla and, if necessary, more milk.

TIPS & TRICKS:

- If you don't like chocolate frosting, try making the cake with buttercream frosting.

BLANCHE'S CHEESECAKE

Carol Harris

"This is Blanche Weisfield's cheesecake recipe, which my mother, Adele Golub, served at many special family dinners. Blanche was a delightful woman who entertained often and elegantly. It is still the lightest cheesecake I have ever tasted. I imagine an update would be to use fresh berries, rather than canned or frozen, for the glaze options."

Serves 12 to 16

Crust:
1½ cups (26-27 wafers) vanilla wafers, crushed
4 tablespoons butter, melted

Butter a 9-inch springform pan.

Combine the wafers and the butter and press the crumbs evenly around the pan.

Filling:
5 eggs, divided
1 cup sugar
16 ounces cream cheese, softened to room temperature
2 cups sour cream
1 teaspoon lemon juice
1 teaspoon vanilla

Preheat the oven to 300°.

Place the egg whites in the bowl of an electric mixer and beat until the whites are stiff. Set aside.

Cream the sugar and cream cheese together in an electric mixer. Add the egg yolks and mix well. Stir in the sour cream, lemon juice, and vanilla. Fold in the beaten egg whites.

Pour the mixture over the crust. Bake for 1 hour and 15 minutes. Turn the oven off and leave the cake in the oven for several hours, or overnight, to cool.

Strawberry Glaze:
1 16-ounce package frozen strawberries
1 tablespoon cornstarch
1 tablespoon sugar

Slowly bring the frozen strawberries to a boil in a small saucepan. Add the cornstarch and sugar and boil for about 5 minutes. Cool, and then pour the glaze over the top of the cooled cheesecake.

Blueberry Glaze:
1 14-ounce can blueberries, with the juices
1 tablespoon cornstarch
1 tablespoon sugar

Separate the juice from the blueberries and place the juice in a small saucepan. Add the cornstarch and sugar to the juice and bring to boil. Boil until thick, add the blueberries, and cool. Pour the glaze over the top of the cooled cheesecake.

DARCY'S CHEESECAKE

Darcy Goodman

"This cheesecake is as dense and rich as they come, but it is easy to make and beautiful to serve with fresh berries on the side."

Serves 12 to 16

Crust:
2 cups graham cracker crumbs
1/2 cup butter, melted

Mix together the graham cracker crumbs and butter. Press the mixture into the bottom of a buttered springform pan.

Filling:
2 pounds cream cheese, room temperature
1 cup sugar
2 eggs
1/2 teaspoon vanilla
1/8 teaspoon almond extract

Cream the cream cheese, sugar, eggs, vanilla, and almond extract. Pour over the prepared crust.

Place the unbaked cheesecake on the middle rack of a cold oven. Then set the heat to 350°. Bake for 35 to 40 minutes from the time you place the cake in the oven. Don't worry if the center isn't set when finished cooking. It will firm up as it cools.

Topping:
2 cups sour cream
1 lemon, juiced
3/4 cup sugar
1/4 teaspoon vanilla
1/8 teaspoon almond extract

While the cake is baking, make the topping by combining the sour cream, lemon juice, sugar, vanilla, and almond extract. Pour the topping over the hot cake and bake for 8 additional minutes, until the sides are bubbling. Remove the cake from the oven and cool on a rack for 2 to 3 hours, until the pan is room temperature. When cool, refrigerate until ready to serve.

TRIPLE CHOCOLATE CHEESECAKE

Julie Faison

"It doesn't get more chocolate-y than this. A wonderful dessert for any occasion!"

Serves 16

Crust:
1½ cups chocolate cookie wafers (about 30), finely crushed
3 tablespoons sugar
⅛ teaspoon cinnamon (optional)
¼ cup unsalted butter, melted

Preheat the oven to 400°.

In a medium bowl, stir together the cookie crumbs, sugar, and cinnamon until blended. Drizzle with the melted butter and mix until well blended and the crumbs are evenly moist. Press the mixture into the bottom of a 9-inch springform pan and about one inch up the sides of the pan.

Bake for 10 minutes and set on a wire rack to cool completely.

Filling:
½ cup sour cream
2 teaspoons vanilla
1 teaspoon instant coffee granules (or espresso powder)
8 ounces bittersweet chocolate, finely chopped
3 8-ounce packages cream cheese, room temperature
3 tablespoons unsweetened cocoa powder, sifted
¼ teaspoon salt
1¼ cups sugar
3 large eggs, room temperature

Mix the sour cream, vanilla, and coffee granules (or espresso powder) in a small bowl. Set aside and stir occasionally until the coffee dissolves.

Melt the chocolate in a double boiler over medium heat (or in a microwave). Stir until smooth and then set aside to cool slightly.

In an electric mixer, beat the cream cheese, cocoa powder, and salt until smooth and fluffy, scraping down the sides of the bowl and paddle often. Add the sugar and continue beating until well blended and smooth. Scrape the melted chocolate into the bowl and beat until blended. Beat in the sour cream mixture until well blended. Add the eggs, one at a time, beating until just blended.

TIPS & TRICKS:

- Don't overbeat the filling once the eggs have been added or the cake will puff up too much during baking.
- To slice, run a thin knife under hot water, wipe it dry, and cut the cake into slices.
- The cheesecake can be frozen by putting the unmolded cake in the freezer until the top is cold and firm, then wrap the cake in two layers of plastic and one layer of foil.

Pour the filling over the cooled crust, smoothing the top.

Reduce the oven temperature to 300° and bake for 50 to 60 minutes, until the center barely jiggles. The cake will be slightly puffed with a few cracks around the edge. Let the cake cool to room temperature on a rack then refrigerate until well chilled, 4 hours to overnight.

When ready to serve, remove the pan's ring and run a long, thin metal spatula under the bottom crust. Carefully slide the cake onto a flat serving plate.

DOUBLE BLACKBERRY PIE

Dani Cone

"Dani Cone has taken the tradition of handing down recipes from one generation to another to a new level, epitomizing the ultimate contemporary 21st century woman. Dani has fond childhood memories of her grandmother, Molly Cone, baking delicious pies, and this is the inspiration behind her current pie business. In 2005, Dani opened her first coffee shop, Fuel, followed by two more in only four years. She has recently opened a brand new bakery called, 'High Five Pie.' Though Dani will not give out her grandmother's original recipes, which, according to Gourmet *magazine, are the 'best in Seattle,' she does share an all-butter crusted, double blackberry pie recipe that she says is very similar to the one she received from her grandmother, Molly. A driven business woman, at work by 4 a.m. daily to bake pies in her commercial kitchen, followed by hands-on management at her pie shops until 8 p.m., Dani is on the fast track as a successful entrepreneur who has been resolute in expanding her love for pie into a rewarding and profitable business. And it all started in her grandmother's kitchen."*

~ Marilyn Kremen

Makes one 9-inch pie

Crust:
2½ cups flour
1 teaspoon salt
1 teaspoon sugar
1 cup unsalted butter, ice cold and cut into ½-inch cubes
¾ cup ice cold water

In a large bowl, combine the flour, salt, and sugar and mix well. Add the butter and mix gently with a pastry cutter, fork, or your hands. Incorporate the butter with the dry ingredients, mixing lightly. The butter pieces should be well-coated in the dry mixture and somewhat flattened out.

Gradually add the cold water, one tablespoon at a time, and continue working until the dough comes together and forms pea-size crumbs. The dough should look like coarse, individual pieces.

With your hands, gather the crumb-like mixture to form the dough into two patties, being very careful not to overhandle the dough. Wrap each patty separately in plastic wrap. Chill for at least 1 hour or up to 3 days.

Filling:
1 cup sugar
3 to 4 tablespoons quick-cooking tapioca
½ teaspoon cinnamon
½ teaspoon nutmeg
6 cups blackberries
3 tablespoons blackberry liqueur or cordial
1 tablespoon lemon juice

Vanilla ice cream, for serving

To make the filling, stir together the sugar, tapioca, cinnamon, and nutmeg in a large bowl. Add the berries, liqueur, and lemon juice and mix gently. Let the mixture stand for 1 hour, stirring occasionally.

Preheat the oven to 375°.

When you are ready to use the dough, remove it from the refrigerator and let it at sit room temperature for 10 minutes to soften, making it more workable. Roll out one piece on a lightly floured surface to fit a 9-inch pie plate. Roll out the second piece of dough so it will fit over the fruit.

Pour the fruit filling into the bottom crust, top with the second top crust, and crimp the edges. Slit the crust in several places so steam can escape. Bake for 35 to 40 minutes, until the top is golden brown. Cool for 30 minutes or bring to room temperature and serve with a good quality vanilla ice cream.

OVER THE TOP PUMPKIN PIE

Leatrice Gutmann

"This was and still is the traditional pumpkin pie for Thanksgiving at our home. It was my mother's, Sally De Leon's, recipe."

Serves 8 to 10

3/4 cup brown sugar
1 envelope unflavored gelatin
1/2 teaspoon salt
1 teaspoon cinnamon
1/2 teaspoon nutmeg
1/4 teaspoon ground ginger
3 eggs, separated
3/4 cup milk
1 1/4 cups canned pumpkin purée
1/3 cup sugar
1 prepared graham cracker pie crust
Whipped cream, as a garnish

In a saucepan, combine the brown sugar, gelatin, salt, cinnamon, nutmeg, and ginger.

Beat the egg yolks in a bowl. Stir the milk into the eggs and add to the saucepan. Over medium heat, cook the mixture, stirring constantly, until it comes to a boil. Remove the pan from the heat and stir in the pumpkin. Let the mixture cool until it mounds slightly when spooned.

Beat the egg whites until soft peaks form. Gradually add the sugar and beat until stiff.

Fold the cooled pumpkin mixture into the beaten egg whites. Pour the filling into the graham cracker crust and refrigerate until firm. Garnish with whipped cream.

CHOCOLATE MERINGUE PIE

Luba Alexander

Serves 6 to 8

3 egg whites
1/2 teaspoon cream of tartar
3/4 cup sugar
3/4 cup pecans, chopped
2/3 cup semisweet chocolate chips
3 tablespoons strong, hot coffee
1 cup whipping cream, whipped

Preheat the oven to 325°.

Beat the egg whites and cream of tartar until stiff, but not dry. Gradually beat in the sugar until the whites are very stiff. Fold in the nuts. Pour into an 8-inch pie plate and bake at for 50 minutes. Cool on a rack.

Melt the chocolate chips. Add the coffee to the melted chocolate, and then gradually add that mixture to the whipped cream. Pour into the meringue shell and refrigerate overnight (or freeze).

TIPS & TRICKS:

- This is great for company as you can make it ahead and freeze it.

CHOCOLATE APRICOT TORTE

Betty Rubenstein

"The tartness of the apricots and the bittersweet chocolate bite in the crust are welcome flavors in this especially-good-in-autumn torte. Be sure to make the filling first, because it needs to cool before spreading over the crust."

Serves 8 to 12

Filling:
11 ounces dried apricots
1½ cups sugar
¾ cup water
3 tablespoons flour
½ lemon, juiced

Combine the apricots, sugar, water, flour, and lemon juice in a heavy saucepan. Bring the mixture to a boil over medium-low heat, stirring frequently. Reduce the temperature and simmer for 20 to 25 minutes, smashing the apricots, until the mixture looks like jam. Remove from the heat and cool completely.

Crust:
3 ounces unsweetened chocolate, roughly chopped
2 cups whole walnuts
1½ cups flour
¾ cup brown sugar, packed
½ teaspoon salt
½ cup butter, chilled and cut into pieces
2 teaspoons vanilla

Preheat the oven to 350°.

Put the chocolate in a food processor, fitted with the steel blade, and chop for 5 pulses. Add the walnuts and pulse a bit more. Then add the flour, brown sugar, salt, butter, and vanilla, and pulse again. When the mixture is well combined (you will see some small chunks of chocolate and nuts), turn approximately two-thirds of the mixture into a 9½-inch springform pan, pressing it about one inch up the side.

Pour the cooled filling on top of the crust. Sprinkle the remaining one-third of the crust mixture on top of the torte.

Bake for about 40 minutes. The crust will brown around the edges.

TIPS & TRICKS:

- The torte can be made a couple of days ahead. Place the prepared crust in the pan, cover, and refrigerate until the torte is ready to bake. The jam can also be made ahead and kept refrigerated until ready to use. Just be sure the jam is at room temperature so it is spreadable before putting onto the crust.

LEAVITT-GOODMAN FAMILY'S FAVORITE ALMOND TORTE

Darcy Goodman

Serve 8 to 10

1¾ cups sliced almonds
¾ cup plus 2 tablespoons powdered sugar
4 large egg whites
¼ teaspoon salt
¾ teaspoon almond extract

Preheat the oven to 325°. Cut a piece of parchment paper to fit the bottom of an 8-inch round nonstick cake pan. Coat the cake pan with cooking spray, put in parchment paper, and spray again.

In a food processor, finely grind 1½ cups of the almonds with ¾ cup of the powdered sugar. Set aside.

Beat the egg whites and salt until soft peaks form. Gradually add the remaining 2 tablespoons of the powdered sugar and continue beating until the egg whites are stiff and glossy. Then beat in the almond extract. Gently fold in the almond mixture in two additions.

Sprinkle the bottom of the pan with the remaining ¼ cup of the almonds. Gently spread the batter into the pan and tap it lightly on counter to remove any air bubbles.

Bake for 40 to 45 minutes, until golden brown and firm in the center. Cool in the pan for 15 minutes, then invert the torte onto a rack. Serve plain, with ice cream, or with berries that have been macerated with a little sugar.

MITZI'S FRUIT KUCHEN

Jane Volinn Preuss

"Some say that cooking is an expression of love. Letters from my Grandmother Mitzi show how my grandmother used food and recipes as a way to reach out to the daughter (Ilse, known as Itte) she loved, who could not cook. Food and cooking, however, clearly reach beyond the food; the recipes show the constant adaptations to the ever-increasing struggle to obtain food and, as such, also reflect the creativity involved in maintaining a life that was not only bearable, but in fact, was worth living. For Grandmother Mitzi, it was a way to mute stress and anxiety while coping with unspeakable horrors as the Nazis tightened the strictures of Jewish life in Vienna. I translated letters from my grandmother Mitzi, which follow this recipe."

Makes one 10- to 11-inch tart

Crust:
1 cup flour
½ cup powdered sugar
½ teaspoon baking powder
½ cup butter, room temperature
2 egg yolks
2 tablespoons Quark, whipping cream, or sour cream
½ lemon, rind grated
1 to 2 teaspoons lemon juice, freshly squeezed

In a food processor, pulse the flour, powdered sugar, and baking powder together 3 times. Add the butter then the egg yolks, one yolk at a time. Add the Quark, and then the lemon zest and lemon juice. Knead the dough into a ball and cool in the refrigerator for about 1 hour. Roll out or press the dough into a 10 or 11-inch pan with removable sides.

Filling:
12 Italian plums
½ lemon, zested and juiced for 1 tablespoon juice
¼ cup sugar
½ teaspoon cinnamon
¼ teaspoon allspice
¼ teaspoon powdered vanilla

Whipping cream or vanilla ice cream, for serving

Preheat the oven to 370°.

Cut the fruit into halves or quarters and lay onto the dough in rows (or a circular pattern if using a round pan). Mix the sugar, cinnamon, allspice, and powdered vanilla. Sprinkle the sugar mixture over the plums.

Bake the kuchen for 10 minutes, then reduce the oven temperature to 350° for 10 minutes, and reduce the oven temperature once more, to 340°, and bake for an additional 10 minutes.

Cool on a wire rack and cut into squares or wedges depending on the pan shape. Serve with whipping cream or vanilla ice cream.

TIPS & TRICKS:

- Instead of plums, try 2 apples, 10 to 12 apricots, or 2 peaches or a combination of fruits. Peel and cut the apples and peaches into 1/8-inch slices.

Letters from My Grandmother Mitzi (translated by Jane Volinn Preuss):
To set the scene, in March 1938, right after the Germans took over Austria, my mother, Itte, left Vienna for Rome. She remained in Italy for one year, until she was able to obtain a visa and a sponsor in the United States. My mother sailed from Naples, Italy, on the *Santorini*, arriving in the U.S. in April 1939. These excerpts are from letters my grandmother Mitzi wrote to my mother between 1939 and 1940.

April 21, 1939
"Today we received your first letter from America and are so happy that you like it so much. Now we would very much like to know how you are getting along. Do you have enough to eat?

"You and Hans [Itte's brother] have experienced and seen so much that we are living through the experiences of our children. You cannot imagine how comforted and happy we are that you are both doing so well.

"I had to let our new help go because we couldn't even let her be near the kitchen where she was absolutely dangerous. She didn't have the foggiest idea of what to do there. Now I always cook first thing; and by 9 in the morning am ready to go. Today I will look for carp; with some things one can always do something, and when it doesn't come out it is not a big loss."

May 5, 1939
"I am naturally so happy with you and that things are going so well and that you are happy. I think how unhappy I was in the past when I could not help you with your problems, but that lies behind us and is forgotten. Your life now is right and smart. In life there is still much that is in the hands of fate, but with a higher power one must trust and hope that everything will come out fine.

June 7, 1939
"We went to the English consulate today to apply for the necessary certification to leave Austria. Then I went to my last cooking class. Last week our cooking instructor demonstrated, then we made dough for the fruit kuchen; you can use either Italian plums or apples, or anything that is in season (see recipe). Now suddenly, Chef Kohn has left and is on the high seas to America where he intends to practice his profession. You might like to call him."

June 10, 1939
"First, I must I say how happy I am that Hans is now booked with the American Line and that in July he will be arriving in America.

"Since you left so much has changed, and almost every moment it changes, again. Since the last 14 days, even to travel in Europe you must go to the consulate to obtain a permit to leave the country. I will tell you that we will stay here as long as possible because we have heard that in other countries people are taking accommodations that are quite unpleasant. By the beginning of next year, if we do not have our permits for America we will then decide where we should go."

July 5, 1939
"With us everything is urgent. We cannot have our visas until our number is issued from Vienna and we are afraid that Austria is like Prague [my grandfather was born in the Czech Republic] and we don't know what to do about it. You cannot believe how hard the goodbyes will be from here. I have so many good friends that to exchange them for a future filled with doubts is hard. Now I must close and make dough for the cherry strudel. It needs to sit for a bit so I will go downtown for some fresh air."

May 14, 1940
"We are getting ready for the move if it is required – we hope it will not be.

"Unbelievably, the cost for a good apple or cherry strudel is now almost nothing, only the filling costs money. You might like to try it in your free time after work."

June 2, 1940
"Itte, how is it going with dinner? Next you could make Wiener schnitzel. You can make it half an hour before guests come and then steam in a covered pot on low flame so that it stays hot and does not dry out. With that, serve potatoes with butter and parsley, which you can steam or put in the oven. Serve with a salad. Since I now cook without help, I have learned a lot and all of my friends have given me recipes that I am putting in a book. Now I have a lot of good and cheap meals and menus and hope that you can use them. One is a wonderful cake with 1 egg; another is stuffed tomatoes – a very tasty vegetable meal!

"A rock has been lifted from our hearts – we just found out we will be able to stay in our apartment."

June 11, 1940
"It is nice to know that you are able to get out into the woods. Itte, you are certainly a smart girl to enjoy yourself over the color of the water from the blue heavens and everything beautiful; others walk right by without noticing such things or they take everything for granted; that is love of life. There is no way to help the kinds of people who take life for granted. You are such a clever girl – although I have never doubted that you are all of these things. So fantastic, wonderful, amazing!"

September 13, 1940
"Yesterday we received your telegram regarding the affidavit. We will send the necessary documents soon."

October 2, 1940
"The cooking expertise is coming along well and I would be very happy if I could bake your favorite things for you. Yesterday our dear cook, Marie, visited and I said to her: through 9 years you have been my misfortune. At first she was astonished at what I said, then Marie smiled as I explained. Because she had always done everything so smoothly I let her do everything—and during that time I forfeited the opportunity to learn. To make up for my past inattention, she has given me some of her recipes."

November 5, 1940
"One of the ladies in the course described a relative who started a shop. I think I would like that – I envision something with cooking. I haven't decided which, but I paint a nice picture about the shop when we are all reunited as a family."

November 12, 1940
"Itte – you shouldn't make so much work out of cooking. I just got a very good, cheap, and fast recipe that you will like. Once a week, make Macaroni or noodles with tomato sauce and Parmesan. First make the noodles. Then for the sauce start with a roux: 3-4 Tbs fat (oil), 3-4 Tbs flour, stir until light yellow (not too dark), add medium size tomato sauce, stir in a few sugar cubes, some salt, then add a little water or soup, bring to a boil. Stuffed peppers are also good and easy."

Ending:
In 1942, my grandmother sent a postcard through the International Red Cross saying: "We are going to the angels." In 1945, when my uncle Hans returned to Europe with the U.S. Army, he went to Vienna. There he found that his parents, Mitzi and Ernst, had been shot on their way to Thereisenstadt Concentration Camp.

BOHEMIAN YEAST DOUGH PLUM CAKE

Steve Adler

"This recipe comes from my mother, Ilse Adler, who learned it from her mother-in-law, and my grandmother, Anna Kohner Adler, who learned it in Bohemia."

Makes one 12x18-inch or two 9x12-inch cakes

2 tablespoons sugar, divided, plus additional for sprinkling
3 to 4 cups flour, sifted
¾ cup milk
½ cup butter, plus extra for greasing the bowl and dough
1½ egg yolks
1 package rapid rise yeast
3 to 5 pounds Italian plums
1 tablespoon unflavored breadcrumbs
Whipped cream (optional)

Mix 1 tablespoon of the sugar into 3 cups of the flour and set aside.

Scald the milk, add the butter to it, and stir until the butter is melted.

Add the milk mixture to the flour mixture and mix thoroughly. Add the egg yolks and mix thoroughly, again. Combine the remaining tablespoon of the sugar and yeast, add them to the flour mixture, and beat with a spoon.

Add the remaining cup of flour to the dough, a little at a time, mixing well, until the dough does not stick to the mixing bowl. Knead the dough by hand until it no longer sticks to your hands or the bowl.

Remove the dough from the bowl and grease the bowl with butter. Return the dough to the bowl, put a little butter on the top of the dough, and cover the bowl with a clean towel.

Turn the oven to 200° for 1 minute then turn it off. Place a dish of hot water in the warm oven, and then put the covered bowl with the dough in the oven. Let the dough rise for 1 hour.

Grease one 12x18-inch baking sheet or two 9x12-inch baking sheets.

Punch the dough down and spread it out with your fingers onto the baking sheet(s); the dough should cover the sheet(s) in a

TIPS & TRICKS:

- If you are serving the cake immediately after cooking, sprinkle granulated sugar over the top and serve it with whipped cream, if desired.

uniformly thick layer. Sprinkle a thin layer of the breadcrumbs over the dough and let it rise again in the oven for 45 minutes to 1 hour.

Preheat the oven to 350°.

While the dough rises, quarter and pit the plums. Place the plums cut-side up in even rows across the dough. Bake for 30 minutes.

TIPS & TRICKS:

- Cake can be cut into 2x4-inch slices and frozen for later use. Defrost in the microwave and sprinkle with sugar before serving.

PLUM CAKE

Doris Stiefel

Makes 15 to 18 servings or two 9-inch cakes

"In Jewish households in Germany before WWII, when plums were in season at the end of summer, freshly baked plum cake was standard fare. The refreshing torte went by various names, depending what part of the country you lived in. My family from Rhineland/Westphalia called it Pflaumenkuchen*; my husband, Ernest's, family from southern Germany knew it as* Zwetschgenkuchen*. No matter the name, we have fond memories of enjoying the cake, often topped with a generous dollop of whipped cream, at afternoon coffee with family and friends, and at Rosh Hashanah. Ernie remembers his mother baking it and also eating it on the balcony at the house of his grandmother. My early memories are of plum cake get-togethers in the garden and warding off the wasps that inevitably were attracted by the sweet aroma of the cake.*

"I learned the recipe from my mother, who together with her sister had learned it from their mother. Who knows how many generations before them had made the same plum confection? The family has spread to all parts of the globe and with it, the tradition of plum cake. Ernie's grandmother in her late seventies made the arduous move to Uruguay, while others came to the U.S.; tragically his parents perished in the Holocaust. My grandparents, after suffering the pogrom of Kristallnacht on November 9, 1938, were able to join their children, who had preceded them to England, where despite bombing and wartime food rationing, the women managed to bake plum cake. Ten years later, my parents and I moved from England to Seattle, and plum cake season continued to flourish here. Naturally, when Ernie and I built our house, we planted a plum tree that has rewarded us with ample crops of Italian plums year after year. Now our grandchildren delight in picking the plums and are clamoring to get the recipe so that they, too, can carry on the plum cake tradition.

"The following recipe is a slightly modified version of the original. I now use a food processor and in keeping with current dietary concerns, I have reduced the fat content in the 'Muerbeteig' pastry; the cake is delicious even without whipping cream."

2 cups flour
5 tablespoons sugar, divided
2 teaspoons baking powder
¾ cup margarine or butter
1 large egg (or liquid egg equivalent)
3 pounds ripe Italian plums, pitted and quartered lengthwise
½ teaspoon cinnamon

Preheat the oven to 375°. Spray an 11x16-inch jelly roll pan with cooking spray.

In a food processor, process the flour, 2 tablespoons of the sugar, and baking powder for 10 seconds. Cut in the margarine or butter and process until finely crumbled. Add the egg and process until the mixture forms a ball around the blade. Press the dough evenly over the bottom of the prepared pan.

Arrange the plums, cut-side up and slightly overlapping, in 6 lengthwise rows on top of the dough. Bake for 20 to 25 minutes, until the crust is golden and the plums begin to juice. Mix the remaining 3 tablespoons of the sugar and cinnamon, and sprinkle the top of the cake with this mixture while the cake is still warm.

TIPS & TRICKS:

- For a 9-inch round cake, cut the recipe in half and arrange plums in concentric circles.

ITALIAN PLUM SHORTBREAD

Carol Starin

"I always make this yummy shortbread torte for Rosh Hashanah – that's because Italian plums are plentiful in the fall. One cold winter day I was riding the elevator at the Summit on First Hill. In the elevator with me was Frieda Sondland – and she was carrying the very same plum cake to one of her neighbors. I turned to her and asked, 'How did you manage to find Italian plums in the middle of the winter?' She told me that she buys the plums in the fall, washes them, cuts them in half, takes out the pits, and freezes them for use all year round. Now why didn't I think of that years ago? One generation tells another."

Serves 8 to 10

2 cups butter
¾ cup sugar, plus more for dipping the plums
4 cups flour
6 tablespoons rum
2 egg yolks
½ teaspoon salt
30 to 40 ripe Italian plums
Powdered sugar, for dusting

Preheat the oven to 450°. Grease a 9x13-inch glass dish for a more torte-like dessert, or a 10x15-ince dish for a thinner, tart-like crust.

For the crust, combine the butter, sugar, flour, rum, egg yolks, and salt until it becomes a thick dough. Press the dough into the prepared baking dish.

Slice the plums in half and remove the pits. Dip the cut sides of plums in sugar, then press them into the dough, cut-side up, in neat rows.

Bake for 15 minutes. Then reduce the oven temperature to 350° and bake for another 30 minutes. Remove and cool. When the torte has cooled, dust it with powdered sugar.

TIPS & TRICKS:

- This can also be made in a 12 or 13-inch round tart pan with a removable bottom.
- Starting in the middle of the dough, overlap the dipped-in-sugar plums in a spiral- fashion, all the way to the edge.

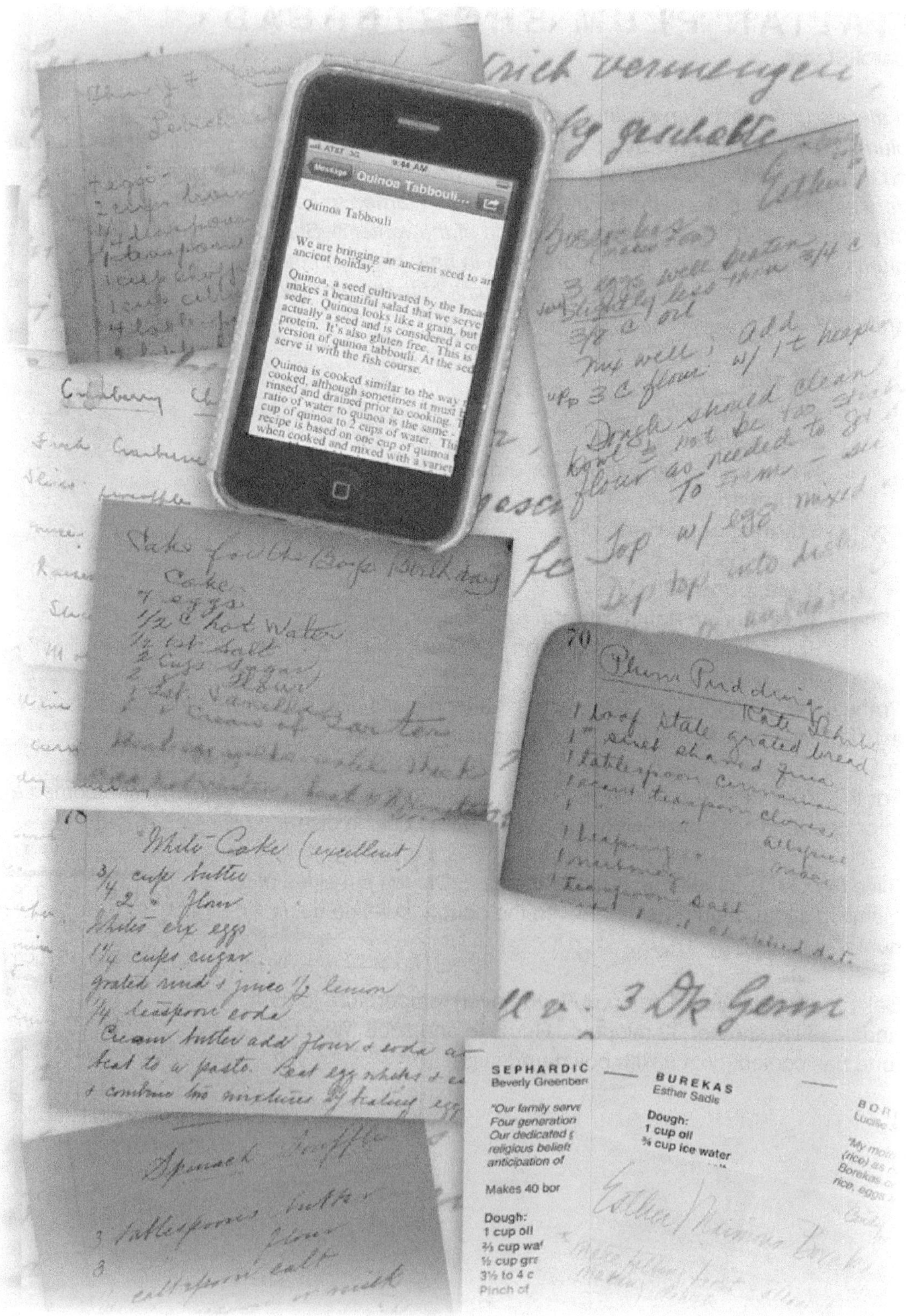
Quinoa Tabbouli
SEPHARDIC
BUREKAS
Esther Sadis
Dough:
1 cup oil
¾ cup ice water
White Cake (excellent)
3/4 cup butter
1¼ cups sugar
Plum Pudding
Cake for the Boys Birthday

Gifts from the Pantry

This chapter is diverse, with recipes for pickles, marinades, sauces, and spreads, from homemade horseradish to hot fudge sauce. A pioneer spirit, both from the old country and the Pacific Northwest, imbues these stories of putting up pickles, scrubbing horseradish root, and grating apples for apple jam.

Who knew how many variations on the pickle could really exist? Judging by our submissions: Tons. Included here are mainly the stories around these pickles, which are as sensory as the taste of the garlicky, briny cucumbers themselves. Gayle Carrol recounts "Pickle Day," the long August day of picking, cleaning, jarring, swimming, and eating as a family, and Cindy Fein Strauss reflects on her childhood, she and her sisters preparing pickles assembly-line style in their big Mount Baker basement. Not only does the salty-dilly taste of the pickles leap off the page, as we read through these memories, we are transported to a late summer day surrounded by extended family.

Toddy Horowitz and Morrene Jacobsen share recipes for Sephardic and Ashkenazi variations on *charoset*, the Passover Seder centerpiece. Dan Asher takes horseradish to a new level, invoking both maven and foodie trends. By getting back to the recipe's roots (literally – he grows the horseradish) and preparing the condiment on his own, some foodies would say he rejects supermarket consumer culture, a very fashionable practice adopted by the "locavore" foodie movement.

A distinct American influence comes through via cranberries, Worcestershire sauce, red wine vinegar, and mustard, as well as through the international flavors from Argentina, Morocco, and Turkey brought here by émigrés.

GIFTS FROM THE PANTRY

"One day my mother was cleaning out some old papers, and she came across my grandmother's pickle recipe. When she showed it to my dad, he got excited, remembering his mother's wonderful pickles. Thinking about the crisp crunch and great taste of the pickles, he decided to make a batch. When the season was right, he went to the market, bought the pickles, dill, and spices, and proceeded to 'put up' the pickles. They were delicious, and from then on my dad became the family pickle man."

~ Luetta Pearl Jermulowske

DILL PICKLES

Gayle Carrol

"The recipe is my mother-in-law's. The family tradition is ours. For about the last 30 years, one Sunday every August has been set aside as 'pickle day.' Our family and our good family friends put up pickles together. Our kitchen is turned into an assembly line. When we started, it was really a day-long activity. We would all go to Remlinger Farms and pick cucumbers. Actually, the grown-ups would pick, and the kids played in the dirt. Our goal was 100 pounds. When we got the cukes home, the wives (and the kids as they got older) would scrub them clean, and the husbands would peel garlic and pack the jars with the cukes, dill, garlic, and spices. By the time this stage was completed, it was lunch time. We would break for lunch and maybe a swim. Then we would return to boil the water and fill the jars. This would take a good part of the afternoon. We would finish late in the afternoon, and there was more swimming and dinner.

"As the years went on, the process has simplified. We buy the cukes from a local produce stand. They are washed in the washing machine. The water is no longer boiled. The garlic cloves come peeled from Costco and the entire process takes about 3 hours. The kids are grown and on their own now, but every year on 'Pickle Day,' they all come back to help."

Makes 1 pound of pickles per 1 quart jar

1 garlic clove
1 tablespoon pickling spice
1 to 3 fresh dill blossoms or one sprig of fresh dill
1 pound of small to medium size pickling cucumbers
1 cup brine, approximately (1 cup non-iodized salt to 20 cups water)

TIPS & TRICKS:

- Cucumbers may be washed in a top-loading washing machine in cold water on gentle cycle. Start washer on small load. Add cucumbers so they have room to move around. Let washer agitate about 3 minutes and drain. Be sure not to let the washer go through a spin cycle as it will bruise the cucumbers.
- The salt can be dissolved in 2 cups of warm water. Then add 18 cups of cold water to measure 20 cups total.
- Try using Ball brand lids and rings.

Clean the cucumbers, being sure to remove any blossom remnants. Boil the lids for one minute in boiling water.

Add the dill to the bottom of each jar. Pack the cucumbers tightly into the jar, staying below the bottom of the mouth. Add the spice and garlic. Add the brine mixture, just covering the cucumbers. Cover with the lid, then seal tightly with the ring.

Store the pickles in a cool, dark location. They will be half-done after approximately one week. To maintain half-done status, store the pickles in the refrigerator. They will keep up to one year.

"My parents, Jane and Midge Fein, were masters at making dill pickles. One of my father's patients had a vegetable stand at the Pike Place Market. Every September, she would have boxes and boxes of pickling cucumbers and heavenly fresh dill for my parents. The five children in our family formed an assembly line in the big basement of our Mount Baker home, washing cucumbers, peeling garlic, packing jars with spices. It took almost a full day, but the pickles we produced were loved by family and friends. I haven't found any pickles since that are as good."

~ Cindy Fein Strauss

"My recipe for dill pickles came from my mother, who showed us her method. For many years my sisters, Bess Leavitt, Edyth Drebin, and I got together for the annual pickle-making – we called it the pickle factory. We would put up between 50 and 100 pounds of cucumbers, giving many jars to friends and family. We would sometimes be joined by our children to wash and sort and stuff cukes in jars. We bought the ingredients from our favorite farmer at the Pike Street Market early in the morning and spent much of the day at our 'factory.'"

~ Isabel Stusser

MOM'S PICKLES

Debra Schwartz, Gail Alexander, and Steve Schwartz

"To fry or not to fry the onions for the chopped liver...
To sprinkle the komishbrot (mandelbreit) with cinnamon or not...
To shake the pickle jar 10 or 12 times, 'with love,' to mix in the salt."

"No matter what the answers, these were the debates that went on in Chehalis, Washington, weekly, monthly, annually. Every time the Schwartz and Cohn families gathered to make their chopped liver, their komishbrot, or their pickles, our grandmother, Esther Schwartz, thought things should be made one way, and her sister, Minnie Cohn, thought they should be made another. And further, both bragged that their way was the most delicious.

"Esther – we called her 'Mom' – and Aunt Minnie arrived in Seattle in 1916 from Brezen, Russian Poland, with their parents, Goldie and David Topolovitz, along with another sister, Pearl, and a brother, Solomon. Their brother, William, was born one year later.

"Minnie Topolovitz met David Cohn. They married and moved to Chehalis in 1927 where Dave opened a furniture store. They introduced Esther to Nate Schwartz, who purchased a men's wear store there. Esther and Nate married and had three children, Ken (our dad), Gloria, and Harold. The three of us and three of our cousins grew up in Chehalis. Aunt Minnie and Uncle Dave never had children of their own, but we were treated like the grandchildren they never had.

"Our family dined together at least once a week with our grandparents, aunt, uncle, and cousins. We all recall those 'family-centric' dinners. Discussions would revolve around local news, national politics, and a wide variety of other topics, but the tie that bound us together as Jews was the preparation and enjoyment of the food. Holiday dinners consisted of chicken soup with matzo balls (custom made for those who preferred light and fluffy or cannonball hard), roasted chicken or brisket, and a kugel. The table would be set with special green, cut crystal glasses, beautiful bone china, and freshly polished silver. On our birthdays, Aunt Minnie and Mom would make 'Cake for the Boys' Birthday,' (page 280) a marvelous sponge cake served with whipped cream.

"We marvel at Mom's and Minnie's ability to do all the food preparation they did without today's modern conveniences of a food processor, microwave, or 24-hour grocery store. Together, we would put up 150 pounds of pickles a year, which would be distributed to relatives and friends throughout the state. Each of those pickle jars needed to be shaken no fewer and no more than 12 times. We would make dozens of pies in one afternoon, and we would make chopped liver for any occasion. Our family always celebrated Hanukah on December 25, and after Schwartz Men's Wear would close for the 'other' holiday on December 24, the whole clan would go to Kit Carson, a local eatery where, although fried chicken livers were not on the regular menu, the restaurant would serve them to us and our extended family. No bread was eaten during Passover, but that was the time of year when

chicken fat made a particularly overwhelming appearance at the holiday table. 'Gribenes,' chicken fat fried until it was crisp, would be sautéed in chicken fat with raw onions.

"Whenever we set our tables now for the holidays or special dinners with Mom's beautiful green glasses, Aunt Minnie's fine china, Sarah Golombeck's (our mother's mother) candelabra, and Mom's linens, we can almost feel the arms of those from generations past wrapped around us. We taste the food and hear the voices telling us, 'Shake the pickle jar exactly 12 times...with love.'"

2 sprigs fresh dill
2 small red chili peppers
2 cloves garlic
8 to 12 pickling cucumbers, farm fresh, small to medium in size
1 tablespoon pickling salt

In a 1-quart jar, place 1 sprig of dill, 1 red pepper, and 1 garlic clove. Pack the pickles in the jar vertically, being careful not to break or bruise them. Add another sprig of dill, another red pepper and another garlic clove. Sprinkle the pickling salt all over. Fill the jar with cold water, screw on the lids, and gently shake "with love" 12 times. Turn the jars 12 times a day for 1 week. Keep the jars in a cool, dark place for one week before serving the pickles.

"The Barde family dill pickle recipe has been in our family for many generations. Our father, Ted Barde, always said that his mother and grandmother were wonderful cooks. Sadly, not too many of their recipes were written down. However, somehow he remembered how to make their dill pickle recipe. He told us that the ladies would always discuss the proper ratio of water to salt.

"As children, we helped make up to 75 jars of dill pickles. We would open a few jars at Rosh Hashanah dinner and rave about how we helped make the pickles. One of us would always throw in an extra hot chili pepper into one or two jars as a joke and a surprise.

"Now the next generation is learning how to make pickles, and we are still quite sure that they are the best pickles we have tasted. They remain a hit at family holidays and year-round."

~ Nina Waldbaum, Amara Rothchild, Lloyd Barde

HORSERADISH

Dan Asher

"I began growing horseradish in order to make Passover gifts for friends and family. Horseradish is easy to grow and simple to prepare. It's the strong smell that becomes the challenge. Rubber gloves and a well-ventilated room are a must. I buy fresh horseradish roots and plant them. In August, I dig up the horseradish and scrub it, peel it, and drop it into a tub of cold water to prevent discoloration."

Makes approximately 1 cup

8 ounces horseradish root, peeled and cubed
¾ cup white vinegar
2 teaspoons sugar
¼ teaspoon salt
Red beet (canned or freshly cooked), grated (optional)

Place the horseradish, vinegar, sugar, and salt in a blender or food processor and pulse until desired consistency. For red horseradish, add a bit of grated red beet.

CHAROSET

Morrene Jacobson

Makes about 5 cups

4 medium Red Delicious apples, peeled and chopped
¾ cup walnuts
2½ tablespoons sugar
2 teaspoons cinnamon
1 lemon, rind grated
4 tablespoons red wine

Combine the apples and nuts in a bowl. Combine the sugar and cinnamon, then fold into the apples. Add the lemon rind and wine and mix well.

TIPS & TRICKS:

- Make a day ahead to give the flavors time to meld.
- I chop the peeled apples in the food processor. The pieces should be small but still distinct pieces, not mushy. I also chop the walnuts (separately) in the food processor, or you can buy chopped walnuts.
- I usually triple the recipe so we have leftovers after the Seder. To do this I make a single recipe 3 times, then combine them all, rather than one big recipe, as it's easier to mix this way.

SEPHARDIC CHAROSET

Toddy Horowitz

"Sephardic Charoset is completely different from that made by Ashkenazi cooks. Over the years, I have found so many who ask how it is made. This is my recipe for Passover Sephardic Charoset."

Makes 4 cups

1 pound pitted dates
2 small Red Delicious apples, unpeeled, cored, and coarsely chopped
½ cup almonds, finely ground
1 cup walnuts, finely ground
¼ cup Passover sweet wine (blackberry or Concord grape)
1 teaspoon vinegar

Place the dates and apples in a saucepan with just enough water to cover the fruit. Bring the water to a boil then lower the temperature to simmer and cook until the fruit is tender. Strain the fruit into a colander, reserving the juice, and set aside.

Pour the fruit mixture into a food processor. Mix in the nuts. Add the wine and vinegar and mix well. If it is too thick, add a little more wine or some of the reserved juices. The mixture should be of spreadable consistency.

APPLE JAM

Nancy Resnik

"Apple Jam is a traditional treat served as the apple dipped in honey for Rosh Hashanah. I also love it on matzos for Passover. Grating and squeezing as much liquid out of the apples as possible, then cooking and stirring the apples in a syrup was always a tedious job. I was visiting an aunt in Istanbul, and she served my favorite – apple jam. The following is her secret to an easy and delicious recipe."

Makes 8 to 10 cups

8 medium to large apples
½ orange
½ lemon
2½ cups sugar
Jars for storing

Peel, core, and grate the apples using a food processor with a metal blade. Gently squeeze the moisture out and place in a large microwavable bowl.

Grind the orange and lemon in a food processor with a steel blade. Add to the apples and mix in the sugar. Microwave the ingredients for 14 minutes. Stir well and microwave for an additional 14 minutes.

Put the apple jam into the jars and refrigerate.

THE BEST HOT FUDGE SAUCE

Karen Hudesman

"This hot fudge sauce recipe was originally printed in the Jewish Day School Cookbook *in 1983, and I continue to make it to this day. My kids loved it, and I have fond memories of them dipping strawberries (and their fingers) in it and loving every bite. It is also delicious over any flavor of ice cream; we used to make designs out of the sauce when adding it to a sundae because it is so thick and smooth. Try drizzling over chocolate cake or in a milk shake."*

Makes about 1½ cups

1 cup sugar
¾ cup water
4 squares unsweetened chocolate
6 tablespoons butter
¼ teaspoon salt
1 egg yolk, well beaten
1 teaspoon vanilla

In a small saucepan over low heat, heat the sugar and water until the sugar dissolves. Add the chocolate, butter, and salt and stir until the chocolate is completely melted. Whisk in the egg yolk and vanilla and whisk until the sauce is smooth and shiny.

TIPS & TRICKS:

- Sauce can be easily and quickly reheated in the microwave for 15 to 30 seconds. Stir, and it will be shiny and smooth.

MARINADE FOR JUST ABOUT ANYTHING

Cindy Masin

"The original recipe called for using this marinade for lamb shish-kebobs, but we have used it to marinate boneless and skinless chicken breasts, sirloin steak, a butterflied-filet roast, and leg of lamb, and every time, with every meat we've grilled, it is fantastic!"

Makes 3½ cups

1½ cups canola oil
¼ cup soy sauce, low-sodium
¼ cup Worcestershire Sauce
2 tablespoons dry mustard
1 teaspoon salt
1½ teaspoons fresh parsley
1 tablespoon ground pepper
½ cup red wine vinegar
1 clove fresh garlic, minced
⅓ cup fresh lemon juice

Blend the oil, soy sauce, Worcestershire Sauce, mustard, salt, parsley, pepper, vinegar, garlic, and lemon juice in a blender for 30 to 40 seconds. Cover and refrigerate until ready to use; will last up to 3 days.

TIPS & TRICKS:

- For chicken and beef, marinate up to 12 hours. For lamb, marinate 24 hours. Grill or cook the chicken, beef, and lamb as you normally would.

MALAGASY PEPPERCORN BUTTER

Elise Topp

Makes 4 cups

"Harry Wong at Trader Vic's gave me this recipe at least 40 years ago. The recipe makes a huge quantity, but can easily be cut in half or even less. Once frozen in a log shape, it can be sliced and defrosted to be used any time to enhance any type of protein."

2 pounds butter (1 pound unsalted, 1 pound salted), softened
2 teaspoons parsley
1 teaspoon dried tarragon
1 teaspoon Dijon mustard
3 cloves garlic, minced
1 4-ounce can Madagascar Green Peppercorns (Poivre Vert)
1 teaspoon brandy
1 teaspoon Worcestershire Sauce
1 teaspoon lemon juice

Mix all the ingredients until smooth, correcting the seasoning and flavoring to taste. Form into 2 logs, 2-inches in diameter, wrap in plastic wrap, and freeze until ready to use. When ready to serve, thaw slightly before cutting the log into ¼-inch slices. Put the desired amount on your choice of protein.

CHIMICHURRI SAUCE

Wendy and Rodrigo Caamano

"Rodrigo is from Argentina where the grilling of meat is taken very seriously. We serve this chimichurri sauce with any grilled meat – beef, lamb, chicken, sausages – all spring and summer long."

1/2 cup olive oil
1/4 cup red wine vinegar
1 small onion, finely diced
1/3 cup parsley or cilantro, finely chopped
4 cloves garlic, finely chopped
1 tablespoon fresh oregano, finely chopped
Salt to taste
1/4 teaspoon cayenne pepper
1/4 teaspoon black pepper, freshly ground

Combine the olive oil, vinegar, onion, parsley (or cilantro), garlic, oregano, salt, cayenne pepper, and black pepper. Mix and let the sauce sit for at least 2 to 3 hours to allow the flavors to develop. Cover and refrigerate until ready to use; will last up to 2 days.

CHARMOULA FOR FISH

Brooke Benaroya Dickson

"This is a variation on the Moroccan sauce charmoula, which is delicious with fish, especially mackerel or sardines. It is also great drizzled on grilled yellow fin tuna, stuffed in a whole fish, or for marinating chunks of halibut for kabobs."

Makes 1½ cups

1 tablespoon cumin seeds
1 bunch cilantro, chopped including some stems with the leaves (about 1 cup)
1 small bunch flat leaf parsley, including some stems with the leaves (about ½ cup)
5 cloves garlic, chopped
1 tablespoon paprika
½ to 1 teaspoon saffron strands
1 medium-hot red chili, seeded and chopped
⅓ to ½ extra virgin olive oil
2 to 3 lemons, zested and juiced
Pinch of salt

Toast the cumin seed and grind in a mortar with a pestle or a spice grinder.

Place the ground cumin, cilantro, parsley, garlic, paprika, saffron, chili, olive oil, zest, and lemon juice in a food processor and blend until mostly smooth. Taste and adjust seasoning.

Cover and refrigerate until ready to use; will last up to 3 days.

CRANBERRY CHUTNEY

Judith Kay

"I chose a recipe that is unusual and something that I make which might be tempting to others. I like it with meat and roasted chicken or turkey, especially because they can be bland. I have also served it alongside a curry dish – made with either chicken or tempeh – which was also great. I love cranberries, so I'll even doctor up my egg whites with it for breakfast."

Makes 4 cups

2 cups fresh cranberries, halved
3 slices canned pineapple, diced
½ cup candied ginger, coarsely chopped
½ cup raisins
½ cup blanched almonds, sliced
1 cup molasses
1 cup wine vinegar
1 teaspoon curry powder
1 teaspoon dry mustard
½ teaspoon ground cloves
1 teaspoon cinnamon
1 teaspoon salt

Mix together the cranberries, pineapple, ginger, raisins, and almonds. Set aside.

Combine the molasses, wine vinegar, curry powder, mustard, cloves, cinnamon, and salt in a large saucepan. Bring to a boil and simmer for about 10 minutes. Add the cranberry mixture, cover, and let stand for several hours.

Glossary

WORD	MEANING
Apio	The botanical name for celery; the root and stalks of this vegetable are cooked with carrots in oil, sugar, and lemon juice until tender.
Bagel	A roll of yeasted dough twisted into a ring that is boiled in simmering water then baked.
Biscocho	A hard, wreath-shaped cookie topped with sesame seeds or cinnamon sugar.
Blintz/Blintzes	Crepe-like pancake often stuffed and rolled with a mixture of cream cheese and cottage cheese.
Boreka	A flakey, pastry turnover in the shape of a half moon, filled with potatoes and cheese, rice, or pumpkin.
Borscht	Cold, sweet and sour beet soup.
Boyikos	Cheese biscuits or crackers.
Boyos	A yeasted, savory pastry filled with spinach and cheese; also sometimes called bulemas.
Burmuelos	Deep fried fritters served at Hanukah with a drizzle of honey and powdered sugar.
Challah	A religiously significant and traditional egg bread served on Shabbat and other Jewish holidays.
Charoset	A mixture of apples, raisins or dates, nuts, and sweet wine served at Passover to represent the mortar used by Jewish slaves in Egypt to build the pyramids.
Charmoula	A marinade of parsley, cilantro, garlic, lemon zest with Moroccan seasonings.
Chimichurri	A sauce of parsley, cilantro, garlic, and olive oil, originating in Argentina and similar to the Moroccan charmoula marinade.
Chulent	A one-pot meal made with meat, beans, and potatoes most often served on Shabbat.

WORD	MEANING
Gefilte Fish	A traditional Jewish delicacy served most often on Shabbat, Passover, and other Jewish holidays. The literal meaning is stuffed fish.
Gribenes	Goose or chicken skin fried in chicken fat with thinly sliced onions until very crisp.
Hamentashen	A three-cornered cookie, filled with filled with fruit, poppy seeds, or chocolate, meant to represent the hat worn by the dreaded Haman, a Persian official who sought the destruction of the Jews.
Hummus	A dip of chickpeas, tahini (sesame paste), garlic, and lemon juice.
Knaidlech	Matzo ball.
Kamishbrot	A nut cookie made from a loaf of dough that has been baked, sliced, then baked again, most closely resembling biscotti, but a bit more crispy.
Kreplach	Meat- or chicken-stuffed pasta that resembles a won-ton.
Knish	A round or sometimes flat pastry, traditionally made with mashed potatoes.
Kuchen	Coffee cake made from a sweet yeast dough.
Kugel	A noodle or potato pudding.
Latke	A potato pancake that is sometimes made with other vegetables.
Mandelbreit	Mandel means almond and breit means bread in this cookie, which is the Eastern European cousin of Kamishbrot.
Marzipan (Massapan)	A candy made from almond paste.
Matzo Brei	Fried matzo.
Meghina	A dish made with ground beef and eggs that is sometimes baked in a crust of matzo and eggs.
Mizrachi	Jews descended from the Jewish Communities of the Middle East, North Africa, and the Caucasus, the region between the Black and Caspian Seas.

WORD	MEANING
Passover	An eight-day Jewish holiday that commemorates the Jews' exodus from Egypt in biblical times.
Parve (Pareve)	A Hebrew term (pareve is the Yiddish term) used to describe food without any meat or dairy ingredients (such as fish, eggs, fruits, and vegetables), which are considered neutral and can be eaten with both meat and milk dishes.
Potchka	To fuss or mess around.
Prakas	Cabbage stuffed with a mixture of meat and rice.
Prasafouchis	Leek patties.
Purim	A festive Jewish holiday that celebrates the deliverance of the Jews by Esther from a planned massacre plotted by Haman.
Quesado	A frittata of eggs, cheese, and vegetables, most often spinach, tomatoes, or zucchini.
Roscas	Rolls made from a yeast dough.
Rugelach	Cinnamon sugar, raisins, jam, or chocolate rolled up in a cream cheese dough and shaped like a crescent.
Schmata	A rag.
Seder	The feast commemorating the exodus of the Jews from Egypt, celebrated on the first two nights of Passover.
Strudel	A thin flakey pastry, filled most often with fruit and nuts, which is then rolled and baked.
Sutlach	Sephardic rice pudding.
Tabouli	Bulgur (cracked wheat) salad mixed with tomatoes and parsley.
Tagine	A slow-cooked stew of vegetables and/or meats; named after the heavy clay pot it is cooked in.
Yapracks or Yaprakies	Grape leaf delicacies filled most often with rice or rice and meat, then rolled up and baked or steamed. The yaprakies most closely resemble Greek dolmas.

Index

C

D

E

F

G

Q

R

S

T

V

W

Y

Made in United States
North Haven, CT
05 November 2026

21760251R00196